SLOW COOKER DOG FOOD COOKBOOK: VET-APPROVED, NUTRITIOUS, AND EASY HOMEMADE RECIPES FOR EVERY BREED

"The ultimate guide to affordable, balanced, and delicious meals for dogs - tailored for busy owners and happy, healthy pets"

ZOEY HARPER

ISBN: 9798303253650

SUMMARY

PREFACE

A note from the author: why cook for your dog

When I started considering the idea of cooking for my dog, my intention was simple: I wanted to do something special for my four-legged best friend. Little did I imagine that this choice would transform not only his life, but also mine. For many of us, dogs are much more than pets; they are family members, faithful companions who give us unconditional love. So why not return that love to them with a healthier, more wholesome and personalized diet?

Cooking for your dog may seem like a demanding task, even a bit overwhelming. I admit that I initially thought so, too. Then I discovered that not only was it doable, but it could also become an enjoyable and rewarding experience. Preparing homemade meals for my dog gave me the confidence that I was nourishing his body with fresh ingredients, free of artificial additives and tailored to his specific needs. Not only that, I had the satisfaction of seeing for myself the benefits of this choice: more energy, a shiny coat, and brighter eyes.

Cooking for your dog is not only a matter of physical health, but also an act of love. This book is my invitation to embark on a journey that will enable you to strengthen the bond with your dog and ensure a longer and happier life for him.

My path to homemade dog food

My adventure began a few years ago when my dog, Max, started suffering from digestive problems. Despite visits to the vet and several brand changes of industrial food, his ailments persisted. It was difficult to watch him suffer, and even more frustrating not to be able to find a solution. One day, talking to a friend of mine who is a pet nutritionist, I discovered home feeding.

At first I was skeptical. I wondered, "Will she really be safe? How can I be sure that Max is getting all the nutrients he needs?" But I was also determined to do my best for him. I started reading books, consulting veterinarians and researching how to create balanced meals. After a few attempts, I saw an improvement in Max's health. His energy had returned, his fur was softer, and most importantly, his digestive problems had disappeared.

The turning point came when I started using the slow cooker. This tool made everything easier: I could prepare nutritious, balanced meals without spending hours in the kitchen. It became a weekly routine: on Sundays I would prepare large quantities of food that I would freeze in portions, ready to be used in the following days. The slow cooker not only saved me time, but also preserved the nutrients in the ingredients, providing healthy and appetizing meals for Max.

This journey has taught me that cooking for our dogs is not an impossible science, but an art accessible to anyone. All it takes is a little initial effort, reliable guidance and a desire to offer something better for our furry friends.

How this book can transform your four-legged friend's health

This book was born out of my personal experience and a desire to share what I have learned along the way. Every recipe, every tip, and every suggestion in these pages is designed to make home feeding simple, safe, and enjoyable for both you and your dog.

Cooking for your dog is not just about mixing a few ingredients and hoping it goes well. It is an act of responsibility that requires awareness and care. This book will guide you step by step, helping you understand your dog's nutritional needs and create balanced meals that will make him feel the best he can be.

A well-fed dog not only lives longer, but lives better. The benefits of fresh, natural food are many: increased energy, better digestive health, a shinier coat, and reduced risk of chronic diseases. In addition, cooking at home allows you to tailor each meal to your dog's specific needs, whether it be intolerances, allergies, or simply taste preferences.

But this book is not just a practical guide; it is an invitation to see your dog as a unique individual with needs and desires that deserve your attention. Every meal you prepare will be an opportunity to strengthen your bond and show him how much you love him.

It doesn't matter if you're a beginner or an expert in the kitchen: with the recipes and tips in these pages, you'll find that cooking for your dog can be a fun and rewarding experience. And with the use of the slow cooker, even busy owners will be able to provide quality meals without sacrificing time and energy.

At the end of this journey, your dog will thank you the way he knows best: with enthusiastic wags of his tail, eyes full of gratitude, and health that speaks for itself. It's a gift you can give him and yourself, and this book will be your guide every step of the way.

INTRODUCTION

The world of home feeding for dogs

Home feeding for dogs is a reality that more and more people are embracing, a way to care for their pets in a conscious and loving way. For many, the decision to prepare homemade meals for their dogs represents an act of caring, a step beyond traditional kibble or packaged wet food. It is a choice that responds not only to the desire to provide the best for our furry friends, but also to the need to tailor their diet to their specific needs.

But what does home-cooked food really mean? And why are so many people abandoning commercial food in favor of home-prepared food? The world of homemade dog food is vast, complex and, at times, fascinating. It offers the opportunity to carefully choose every ingredient that goes into your dog's bowl, ensuring quality, freshness and preparation free of chemical additives, preservatives and by-products.

One of the main motivations for owners to choose homemade food is the growing awareness about the limitations of industrial food. Although many commercial products are well balanced nutritionally, they do not always offer the necessary transparency about what they actually contain. This can be a problem for dogs with special allergies, intolerances, or sensitivities. Preparing meals at home allows you to know exactly what you are offering your dog, prioritizing fresh, nutritious ingredients.

Furthermore, home feeding is not a standard solution-it can be adapted to each dog, taking into account its age, breed, level of physical activity, and health condition. For example, an active puppy will have different nutritional needs than an older dog with joint problems, and a large dog will need different portions and proportions than a small Chihuahua. This flexibility is one of the great advantages of cooking at home.

Another key aspect of home feeding is the bond that is created between you and your dog. Preparing meals with care is a loving gesture that strengthens your relationship with your four-legged friend. It is a way of telling him, "I care about your health and well-being." This bond, made up of attention and shared moments, enriches daily life and creates an even deeper relationship.

Of course, like any change, moving to home feeding requires commitment and awareness. It is not simply a matter of putting together a few ingredients and hoping for the best. It is important to understand the specific nutritional needs of dogs and ensure that each meal is balanced and safe. Working with your veterinarian or a specialized nutritionist is essential to ensure that your dog gets all the nutrients he needs.

Then there is the practical aspect: cooking for your dog does not have to become an onerous or complicated task. With tools like the slow cooker, you can make the process simple and efficient, preparing large quantities of food at once and storing it for the next few days. This preparation mode saves time without compromising food quality.

Finally, choosing homemade food also means taking a step toward greater sustainability. By using local, seasonal, quality ingredients, you can help reduce the environmental impact associated with the production and transportation of commercial pet food.

The world of home feeding for dogs is, therefore, a universe of possibilities. It is a way to take care of your dog's health and well-being, to build a deeper bond, and to make informed and responsible choices. This book is here to guide you on this journey, giving you the knowledge and tools you need to start with confidence and peace of mind. With the right approach, you will discover that cooking for your dog is not only an act of caring, but also an experience that will enrich the lives of both of you.

Why homemade food is an excellent choice

Preparing food for your dog at home is an option that is gaining more and more popularity, not only because of the benefits it offers our furry friends, but also because of the peace of mind and control it gives us owners. It is an option that combines love, attention and a dash of creativity, turning the simple act of feeding your dog into a real act of conscious care.

One of the main advantages of homemade food is the ability to customize each meal to your dog's specific needs. Each animal has unique needs, influenced by factors such as age, breed, physical activity level, and health conditions. With home feeding, you can create tailored meals, ensuring that they are balanced and tailored to your four-legged friend's individual needs. This is especially important for dogs with allergies, intolerances or digestive disorders, situations in which commercial food may not offer adequate solutions.

Another key aspect is the quality of ingredients. When you cook for your dog, you have full control over what you put in the bowl: you can choose fresh foods that are free of preservatives, artificial coloring, and poor-quality by-products often found in many industrial foods. This not only improves the nutritional quality of the meals, but also reduces the risk of exposure to substances potentially harmful to your dog's health.

Homemade food also offers the advantage of transparency. There are no difficult-to-decipher labels, endless lists of ingredients, or additives with complicated names. You know exactly what you are offering your dog and can feel confident about the choice you have made. This clarity translates into greater peace of mind for you and better well-being for your dog.

Nutritionally, homemade food can contribute significantly to your dog's overall health. A fresh, natural diet, when well balanced, supports digestion, improves skin and coat health, strengthens the immune system, and helps maintain a healthy weight. Many owners also report an improvement in their dog's energy and behavior after switching to a home diet.

There is also an emotional aspect that should not be underestimated. Preparing meals for your dog is an act of love that reinforces the special bond you share. Every time you devote yourself to cooking for him, you are showing your commitment and care, and your dog senses this attention. It is not uncommon to see a dog wagging his tail enthusiastically as he watches his owner prepare food!

Another reason homemade food is an excellent choice is its flexibility. You can adapt the recipes to the seasons, taking advantage of fresh, seasonal ingredients, or vary the meals to keep your dog interested and satisfied. You can also include superfoods and particularly nutritious ingredients that support long-term health.

Finally, cooking for your dog can be a rewarding experience for you as well. It is not only an opportunity to improve your pet's life, but also to acquire new skills and healthy habits. Many owners find that by starting to cook for their dog, they also pay more attention to their own nutrition, creating a healthier lifestyle for the whole family.

Home feeding is not just a way to feed your dog: it is an opportunity to care for him in a deeper and more conscious way. It doesn't matter if you are a beginner or already experienced: with the right approach and reliable guidance, you can turn your dog's meals into a time of well-being and love that will last a lifetime.

Dispelling myths about canine nutrition

When it comes to canine nutrition, we often come across myths and misconceptions that can confuse even the most careful owners. These clichés, often passed down over time without real scientific basis, can negatively influence nutritional choices for our four-legged friends. It is important to distinguish between research-based facts and unfounded beliefs to ensure a healthy and balanced diet for our dogs. In this section we will dispel some of the most common myths about canine nutrition.

Myth 1: Dogs must eat only kibble to be healthy

One of the most entrenched myths is that dogs can be fed exclusively kibble to stay healthy. Although high-quality kibble is a practical and balanced option for many owners, it is not the only viable choice. Homemade food, if well planned, can offer the same nutritional benefits, with the advantage of using fresh ingredients and no artificial additives. In fact, many veterinarians and pet nutritionists agree that a varied diet that includes fresh, natural foods can improve a dog's overall well-being.

Myth 2: Table scraps are always harmful to dogs

It is true that some human foods are dangerous for dogs, such as chocolate, onions and grapes, but not all table scraps are harmful. Many foods we consume regularly, such as chicken cooked without seasonings, brown rice, carrots or sweet potatoes, can be perfectly safe and even beneficial for dogs. The key is knowing which foods are suitable and offering them in the right amounts. Turning healthy leftovers into balanced meals is a sustainable and healthy practice, but it should always be done with awareness.

Myth 3: Raw meat is dangerous for dogs

Raw meat feeding, known as the BARF (Biologically Appropriate Raw Food) diet, is a controversial topic.

Some argue that it is dangerous because of the risk of bacterial contamination or parasites, while others believe it is the most natural choice for dogs, being carnivores by nature. The truth lies in the middle: a raw meat diet can be safe and nutritious if prepared and managed properly, using quality meat and following strict hygiene standards. However, it is not suitable for all dogs or all owners. As always, it is essential to consult a veterinarian before embarking on this type of diet.

Myth 4: Dogs cannot eat vegetables or carbohydrates

Another common myth is that dogs, being descendants of wolves, must eat meat exclusively. Although animal protein is an essential component of their diet, dogs are not obligate carnivores, but opportunistic omnivores. This means they can digest and benefit from a variety of foods, including complex carbohydrates such as rice, oats and potatoes, as well as vegetables such as carrots, zucchini and spinach. These foods provide fiber, vitamins, and minerals that contribute to their overall well-being.

Myth 5: Dogs don't need supplements if they eat homemade food

Many owners think that preparing homemade meals is sufficient to meet all of their dog's nutritional needs. However, a homemade diet does not always provide the right balance of essential nutrients such as calcium, phosphorus or omega-3 fatty acids. Supplements can be helpful in filling any nutritional gaps, especially if regular meals are prepared without the assistance of a nutritionist. Again, it is essential to consult your veterinarian to identify the most suitable supplements.

Myth 6: Industrial foods are always harmful

Not all industrial foods are the same. There are excellent quality products that offer complete and balanced nutrition designed to meet the specific needs of dogs. The problem arises with low-quality foods, which are often full of fillers, artificial preservatives and meat by-products of dubious origin. The important thing is to know how to read labels and choose reliable products, avoiding unfounded generalizations.

Myth 7: All dogs can eat the same diet

Every dog is unique and has specific nutritional needs that depend on factors such as age, breed, weight, physical activity level, and health condition. Thinking that there is a universal diet suitable for all dogs is a common mistake. For example, a growing puppy requires more protein and calcium than an older dog, while a dog with kidney problems may need a diet low in protein. Personalizing your dog's diet is critical to ensuring a long and healthy life for your dog.

Dispelling these myths is the first step in building a more informed understanding of canine nutrition. Feeding your dog is not just about filling a bowl, but making informed choices that respect his or her individual needs. A balanced diet that combines scientific knowledge and quality ingredients can significantly improve your dog's health and well-being. With the right information, you can overcome clichés and give your four-legged friend the best he deserves.

The benefits of cooking with a slow stove

In recent years, the slow cooker has become one of the most beloved tools in kitchens around the world, and not just for preparing meals for humans. This versatile and practical appliance has also proven to be a valuable ally for those who want to cook healthy and nutritious meals for their dogs. But why choose a slow cooker to prepare food for your four-legged friend? The benefits are many and go far beyond mere convenience.

1. Conservation of Nutrients

One of the main advantages of the slow stove is its ability to cook food at a low temperature for long periods of time. This method preserves essential nutrients in ingredients, such as vitamins, minerals, and antioxidants, which can be lost with other high-temperature cooking methods, such as boiling or frying. For dogs, who depend on a balanced diet to stay healthy, this is critical. Vegetables remain rich in vitamins, animal proteins retain their nutritional quality, and starches, such as potatoes and rice, are also more easily digested.

2. Ease of Preparation

The slow cooker is perfect for those who have busy lives but still want to provide their dog with homemade meals. Once you have selected and prepared the ingredients, all you have to do is put them in the slow cooker, set the timer, and let the device do the rest. This saves you valuable time by not having to follow every step of the cooking process. You can engage in other activities or spend time with your dog while his meal slowly prepares.

3. Homogeneous and Safe Cooking

The slow cooker's slow, even cooking ensures that all ingredients are cooked to perfection, reducing the risk of raw or undercooked portions that could be harmful to the dog's health. In addition, the constant and controlled temperature eliminates any bacteria or parasites in the raw food, making the meal safe without compromising its nutritional value.

4. Simplicity in Creating Balanced Meals.

With the slow cooker, it is easier to prepare balanced recipes that combine protein, carbohydrates and vegetables in the right proportions. Thanks to the long cooking time, the flavors of the ingredients blend better, creating appetizing meals for even the pickiest dogs. It is also an excellent way to include nutritious ingredients, such as lentils, oats, or sweet potatoes, that might require longer cooking times with other methods.

5. Reducing Food Waste

Another great advantage of the slow cooker is the ability to use ingredients that might otherwise be discarded. Less valuable pieces of meat, vegetable scraps, and other parts we don't usually use in our recipes can be turned into nutritious meals for your dog. This not only reduces waste but is also a way to save money without compromising food quality.

6. Energy Saving.

The slow cooker uses less energy than a traditional oven or a stove that is on for several hours. This makes it an environmentally friendly and economical choice for those who want to cook regularly for their dog. It also does not produce excessive heat, making it ideal for cooking even during the hottest months.

7. Increased Appetite for Dogs.

Slow cooking food intensifies the natural flavors of the ingredients, making meals more palatable for dogs. Even the pickiest dogs or dogs with difficult appetites often find food prepared in a slow cooker irresistible. This can be especially helpful for older or sick animals who may have lost interest in food.

8. Flexibility in Recipes

The slow cooker allows you to experiment with different ingredients and combinations to suit your dog's specific needs. You can customize each recipe according to his preferences or your veterinarian's directions. For example, if your dog needs a low-fat diet, you can use lean meat and low-calorie vegetables. If, on the other hand, he requires a higher caloric intake, you can include energy-rich ingredients such as brown rice or quinoa.

9. Ideal for Preparation in Batches

The slow cooker is perfect for preparing large quantities of food at once, which you can then divide into portions and store in the refrigerator or freezer for the next few days. This practice not only saves you time, but ensures that your dog always has healthy meals ready to serve, even on busy days.

10. A Sustainable and Practical Routine

Finally, cooking with a slow stove can become a sustainable and practical routine that is easily integrated into your daily life. It is a tool that allows you to take care of your dog without adding undue stress or commitment to your day. Over time, you may find that this simple appliance becomes one of your most valuable allies, not only for cooking, but also for strengthening the special bond with your dog.

In conclusion, the slow cooker is not just an appliance, but a means to ensure healthier, safer and tastier meals for your dog. It is a choice that simplifies your life, improves his and turns mealtime into a time of mutual care and well-being.

1. UNDERSTANDING YOUR DOG'S NUTRITION

THE NUTRITIONAL BASICS: PROTEINS, FATS, CARBOHYDRATES AND MICRONUTRIENTS

To ensure your dog's healthy and active life, it is essential to understand the basics of canine nutrition. Every dog is unique, but there are universal nutritional principles that can guide you in preparing balanced meals. Protein, fat, carbohydrates, vitamins and minerals are the basic building blocks of every dog's diet. These nutrients work together to support bodily functions, provide energy, and keep your four-legged friend at peak health.

Protein: The foundation of canine health

Protein is the cornerstone of a dog's diet. They are essential for growth, tissue repair, maintenance of muscle mass, and production of enzymes and hormones. Proteins are made up of amino acids, some of which are essential, which means the dog must get them directly from food because his body cannot produce them on its own.

High-quality protein sources include:

- **Meat**: Chicken, turkey, beef and lamb.
- **Fish**: Cod, salmon and sardines, which also offer omega-3 fatty acids.
- **Eggs**: An excellent source of easily digestible protein.

- **Legumes**: Lentils and chickpeas, useful for enriching a balanced diet.

The amount of protein needed depends on the dog's age, activity level and overall health. Puppies, for example, need more protein than adult dogs because they are growing rapidly. Older or sick dogs can also benefit from a diet rich in high-quality protein, as long as their veterinarian approves.

A common mistake is to believe that "more protein" automatically means "more health." However, too much can put a strain on a dog's liver and kidneys, especially if there is pre-existing disease. Balancing the quantity and quality of protein is therefore essential.

Fats: The main source of energy

Fats are not only a concentrated source of energy, they also play a crucial role in the health of a dog's coat, skin and joints. They provide essential fatty acids, such as omega-3 and omega-6, which are critical for reducing inflammation, supporting the immune system, and promoting a healthy appearance.

Common sources of healthy fats include:

- **Fish oil**: Rich in omega-3, especially useful for dogs with joint problems or inflammation.
- **Chicken fat**: A natural and easily digestible source.
- **Flaxseed**: Rich in omega-3s and fiber.
- **Coconut oil**: An easily metabolized fat that can improve skin and coat health.

It is important to note that fats, although essential, should be offered in moderation. An excess can lead to obesity, which is a risk factor for numerous diseases, including diabetes and joint problems. Similarly, a deficiency in fats can cause dry skin, dull coat and reduced immune function.

Carbohydrates: Sustainable Energy

Carbohydrates are not essential in a dog's diet, but they can be a useful source of energy, especially for active dogs. They also provide fiber, which is essential for healthy digestion. It is important to choose complex, whole-grain carbohydrates, which release energy gradually and help keep blood sugar levels stable.

Healthy sources of carbohydrates include:

- **Brown rice**: Easy to digest and rich in fiber.
- **Sweet potatoes**: A source of complex carbohydrates and beta-carotene.
- **Oats**: A highly digestible food rich in soluble fiber.
- **Quinoa**: A gluten-free pseudo-cereal, rich in protein and carbohydrates.

Not all carbohydrates are suitable for dogs. Corn, for example, is often used in industrial foods as a filler, but it has low nutritional value. Similarly, white bread and other refined foods should be avoided.

Micronutrients: Vitamins and minerals

Vitamins and minerals are the invisible but indispensable nutrients in your dog's diet. They support every function of the body, from bone growth to immune system health to nervous functioning and blood clotting.

Essential vitamins:

- **Vitamin A**: Essential for vision, growth and skin health. Found in carrots and sweet potatoes.
- **Vitamin D**: Helps in calcium absorption and maintenance of bone health. Can be supplemented through fish.
- **B vitamins**: Important for energy metabolism. Found in meat, eggs, and whole grains.
- **Vitamin E**: A powerful antioxidant that protects cells from damage. It is found in seeds and vegetable oils.

Basic minerals:

- **Calcium and phosphorus**: Essential for healthy bones and teeth. A common source is pulverized bone (well cooked and safe) or eggs.
- **Zinc**: Promotes healthy skin and hair. It is found in meat and pumpkin seeds.
- **Iron**: Supports the formation of red blood cells. It is present in red meat and green leafy vegetables.

An important aspect to consider is that an excess or deficiency of vitamins and minerals can be harmful. For example, too much calcium can cause joint problems in growing puppies, while an iron deficiency can lead to anemia. Working with a veterinarian or specialized nutritionist is essential to find the right balance.

The importance of water

Although often overlooked, water is the most important nutrient in your dog's diet. It accounts for about 60-70 percent of body weight and plays a key role in almost every physiological function, from nutrient transport to body temperature regulation. Make sure your dog always has access to fresh, clean water, especially if he is on a home diet or eats dry food.

Understanding the nutritional basics is the first step in ensuring a balanced and healthy diet for your dog. Protein, fats, carbohydrates and micronutrients work together to support your four-legged friend's body and mind, improving his quality of life. Every dog has unique needs, so it is important to tailor his diet to suit his characteristics and consult a veterinarian or pet nutritionist for personalized advice. With the right knowledge, you can give your dog the food he or she deserves: nutritious, balanced, and lovingly prepared.

THE SIZE OF THE DOG: A DETERMINING FACTOR

The size of the dog is the first element to consider when setting portions. Small dogs, such as chihuahuas, have different caloric needs than large dogs, such as golden retrievers or German shepherds. This is because smaller dogs generally have a faster metabolism and require a greater amount of calories per pound of body weight than large dogs.

- **Small** dogs: These dogs, who often weigh less than 10 kg, require smaller but energy-rich meals. It is important to choose nutrient dense foods, as their stomachs are smaller and cannot hold large volumes of food.

- **Medium-sized dogs**: They weigh between 10 and 25 kg and have intermediate caloric needs. Their portions should be balanced to provide sufficient energy without overdoing it, especially if they lead a less active lifestyle.

- **Large or giant** dogs: These dogs, weighing over 25 kg, require more generous portions, but care must be taken not to overdo the calories. Being overweight can put a strain on the joints and cardiovascular system.

A common mistake is to think that a large dog automatically needs more food than a small one. In reality, calorie needs depend not only on size but also on other factors, such as activity level and individual metabolism.

Race: An important indicator

A dog's breed can influence the type and amount of food needed. Some breeds, such as Labrador retrievers, tend to gain weight easily and require more controlled portions. Others, such as border collies or greyhounds, are naturally active and require more calories to support their dynamic lifestyles.

In addition, some breeds have specific needs. For example:

- French bulldogs may have digestive problems and benefit from smaller, more frequent meals.
- Nordic dogs, such as Siberian huskies, have efficient metabolisms and may need less food than breeds of similar size.
- Dachshunds, with their elongated conformation, require strict weight control to avoid back problems.

Understanding the characteristics of your dog's breed is essential to properly calibrate portions.

Lifestyle: Active or sedentary?

Your dog's lifestyle plays a crucial role in determining portion sizes. A dog that spends most of the day resting has lower caloric needs than one that goes for long walks, runs or plays sports.

- **Very active dogs**: Dogs that participate in sports such as agility or accompany their owners on hikes need a higher caloric intake. This is because they burn more energy throughout the day and need food that supports their dynamic lifestyle.

- **Moderately active dogs**: Most dogs fall into this category. They take regular walks but are not particularly active. For them, it is important to maintain a balance between calories consumed and calories burned.
- **Sedentary** dogs: Older dogs or those leading quiet lives require fewer calories to avoid weight gain. Portions should be reduced, but without sacrificing nutritional balance.

Other factors to consider

In addition to size, breed, and lifestyle, there are other elements to consider when calibrating portions:

- **Age**: Growing puppies require more energy and nutrients than adults, while older dogs may require fewer calories but easier-to-digest foods.
- **Health conditions**: Dogs with health problems, such as diabetes or arthritis, may need specific diets that include calibrated portions to support treatment of their conditions.
- **Reproductive status**: Spayed or neutered dogs tend to have a slower metabolism and may need slightly reduced portions.

How to determine the correct portions

A practical way to start is to calculate your dog's daily caloric needs. This can be done using a basic formula:

1. Determine your dog's ideal weight (in kg).
2. Multiply the weight by a factor that varies with activity level:
   - Sedentary dogs: 30 x body weight (kg) + 70
   - Moderately active dogs: 40 x body weight (kg)
   - Very active dogs: 50 x body weight (kg)

This formula will give you an estimate of the daily calories needed. Once you know this value, you can divide the calories between meals, taking into account the energy density of the foods you are offering.

Adjusting portions over time

Your dog's dietary needs may change over time. It is important to regularly monitor his weight, activity level, and overall health status to make any changes. For example, if you notice that your dog is gaining weight, you may need to reduce portions slightly or increase physical activity. Similarly, if he seems lethargic or hungry after meals, he may need more caloric intake.

Calibrating portions according to your dog's size, breed and lifestyle is a process that requires observation, attention and a bit of flexibility. There are no rigid rules, but with an understanding of your dog's specific needs and the support of a veterinarian, you can ensure that he is getting the right amount of food to live a long and healthy life. Remember, a balanced diet is the first step toward your four-legged best friend's well-being.

FOOD ALLERGIES, INTOLERANCES AND SENSITIVITIES

Nutrition is an essential component of dogs' health and well-being, but not all foods are suitable for every individual. Just as with humans, dogs can develop allergies, intolerances, or food sensitivities, which can negatively affect their quality of life. Understanding the difference between these conditions, recognizing their symptoms, and knowing how to manage them is critical to providing your dog with a diet that not only nourishes him, but helps him live better.

The difference between allergies, intolerances and sensitivities

People often use the terms "allergy," "intolerance," and "sensitivity" as synonyms, but these are distinct conditions with different causes and manifestations.

- **Food allergies**: This is a reaction of the immune system to a protein in a food. The body mistakenly identifies this protein as a threat and triggers an immune response, which can manifest as skin, gastrointestinal or respiratory symptoms. Food allergies are relatively rare in dogs, but when they occur they can be chronic and difficult to manage.

- **Food intolerances**: Unlike allergies, intolerances do not involve the immune system. They occur when the dog cannot properly digest a specific food or component, such as lactose in dairy products. Symptoms are often limited to the digestive system, such as diarrhea, bloating or cramping.

- **Food sensitivities**: This term covers a broader range of nonspecific reactions that can include both digestive symptoms and other disorders. Sensitivities can be difficult to identify because symptoms can be intermittent and not linked to a single food.

Common symptoms of eating problems

Symptoms of food allergies, intolerances or sensitivities may vary from dog to dog, but there are common signs to watch for:

- **Skin symptoms**: Persistent itching, hair loss, reddening of the skin, dermatitis or recurrent ear infections. These symptoms may be localized (such as on the paws or around the muzzle) or widespread.

- **Gastrointestinal problems**: Vomiting, diarrhea, flatulence and abdominal bloating are signs that the dog's digestive system may not tolerate a particular food.

- **Respiratory symptoms**: Although rarer, some dogs with food allergies may present with sneezing, coughing or difficulty breathing.

- **Behavioral alterations**: Chronic discomfort caused by an allergy or intolerance can lead to changes in behavior, such as irritability, lethargy, or apathy.

Most common causes of food reactions

Food reactions in dogs are often related to certain ingredients commonly found in industrial foods or home diets. Some of the main "culprits" include:

- **Animal protein**: Chicken, beef, lamb, pork, and fish are common sources of food allergies because they contain proteins that can trigger an immune response.
- **Grains**: Although dogs are generally able to digest grains, some may develop intolerances to wheat, corn or soy.
- **Dairy**: Many dogs are lactose intolerant, which means they cannot properly digest products such as milk, cheese or yogurt.
- **Additives and preservatives**: Some chemical additives or preservatives found in low-quality dog food can cause food sensitivities.

How to identify a food problem

If you suspect that your dog has a food allergy, intolerance, or sensitivity, the first step is to carefully monitor the symptoms and consult a veterinarian. Your veterinarian may suggest one or more of the following approaches:

- **Elimination** diet: This method involves removing all suspicious foods from the dog's diet and gradually introducing individual ingredients to identify which is causing the reaction. The elimination diet requires time and patience, but it is one of the most effective ways to identify allergens.
- **Allergy** testing: There are specific tests that can help determine whether the dog is allergic to certain foods, but these tests are often less accurate than the elimination diet.
- **Observation of changes**: Noting any improvement or worsening in the dog's symptoms during the feeding transition can provide useful clues.

Management of allergies and intolerances

Once the problem is identified, the next step is to adapt your dog's diet to avoid the triggering ingredient and provide a balanced diet. Here are some tips for managing food allergies and intolerances:

- **Choose simple** ingredients: Offer meals with few ingredients to reduce the risk of reactions.
- **Opt for alternative proteins**: If your dog is allergic to chicken, for example, you can try less common proteins, such as rabbit, duck or venison.

- **Exclude processed foods**: Low-quality commercial dog foods often contain fillers, additives and by-products that can aggravate food sensitivities.
- **Include hypoallergenic** foods: Some foods, such as brown rice, sweet potatoes, and white fish, are generally well tolerated and can be a safe foundation for your dog's diet.

Home diet for dogs with dietary problems

For dogs with allergies or intolerances, a homemade diet can be the ideal solution. Preparing food at home allows you to control exactly what you put in your dog's bowl, eliminating any suspect ingredients.

Here are some suggestions for creating a balanced home diet:

- **Consult a veterinarian or animal nutritionist**: It is essential to ensure that the home diet is balanced and contains all the necessary nutrients.
- **Vary ingredients**: Even dogs with allergies benefit from a varied diet, as long as the foods are safe.
- **Monitor portions**: Portions should be appropriate for the dog's caloric and nutritional needs.

Preventing future reactions

Even if your dog has already developed allergies or intolerances, there are some strategies to prevent further problems:

- **Introduce new foods gradually**: When trying new ingredients, add them one at a time and observe any reactions.
- **Avoid potentially problematic** foods: Reduce exposure to foods rich in preservatives, additives or artificial coloring.
- **Provide a balanced diet**: A rich and varied diet can help strengthen your dog's immune system, reducing the risk of developing new sensitivities.

Food allergies, intolerances, and sensitivities may seem like complex challenges, but with the right knowledge and attention, they can be managed effectively. Knowing the symptoms, identifying the causes and adapting your dog's diet will allow you to significantly improve his quality of life. Remember, your dog's well-being begins in the bowl: with food prepared with love and awareness, you can make a difference in his daily health and happiness.

THE IMPORTANCE OF VETERINARY APPROVAL

When it comes to feeding your dog, every decision has a direct impact on his or her health and well-being. This is even more true for those who decide to go the home feeding route, which, while offering more control over the quality of ingredients, requires a deep understanding of the dog's nutritional needs. This is where the importance of veterinary approval comes in. Consulting a veterinarian before making significant changes to your dog's diet is not only a good practice, but an essential step in ensuring that your four-legged friend receives the best.

Why the veterinarian is essential

Your veterinarian is your primary ally when it comes to caring for your dog. His or her training, knowledge, and experience allow him or her to assess your dog's overall health and identify any problems that might affect feeding. Although much information is easily accessible online, every dog is unique, and only a professional can provide personalized guidance based on your pet's specific needs.

1. Understanding of individual nutritional needs

Each dog has different nutritional needs, influenced by factors such as:

- **Age**: Puppies need energy- and nutrient-rich diets to support growth, while older dogs might benefit from low-calorie foods to prevent obesity.
- **Size and breed**: Large breeds may have different needs than small breeds, both in terms of calories and specific nutrients such as calcium.
- **Lifestyle**: An active dog will need more energy than a sedentary one.
- **Health conditions**: Diseases such as diabetes, kidney failure, or food allergies require individualized diets.

Only a veterinarian can evaluate all these aspects and suggest a food plan that takes into account your dog's particular needs.

2. Preventing nutritional deficiencies or excesses

Home feeding offers the advantage of knowing exactly what you are giving your dog, but it also carries the risk of creating an unbalanced diet. For example, a calcium deficiency can cause skeletal problems, while an excess of vitamin A can lead to toxicity. Your veterinarian, often in conjunction with an animal nutritionist, can help you balance nutrients properly, making sure the diet is complete and appropriate for your dog.

Recognizing warning signs

Even the most alert owners may not immediately notice signs of distress or problems caused by inadequate nutrition. Your veterinarian can detect early signs of malnutrition or other feeding complications during routine checkups. These may include:

- **Changes in skin and hair**: Loss of shine or the appearance of itching may indicate a deficiency of essential fatty acids or vitamins.

- **Digestive problems**: Vomiting, diarrhea or bloating may be symptoms of an unsuitable diet.
- **Weight fluctuations**: Unexplained weight gain or loss could result from inadequate caloric intake or a metabolic problem.

Early intervention by your veterinarian can prevent these problems from worsening, improving your dog's quality of life.

Management of specific health conditions

For dogs with pre-existing conditions, veterinary approval becomes even more crucial. Here are some examples where veterinary supervision is essential:

- **Kidney failure**: Dogs with kidney problems require diets low in protein and phosphorus to reduce the strain on the kidneys.
- **Diabetes**: A diet with a low glycemic index can help keep blood sugar levels stable.
- **Gastrointestinal problems**: In case of colitis or intestinal sensitivity, your veterinarian may suggest specific easily digestible foods.
- **Food allergies and intolerances**: Your veterinarian can guide you in choosing safe and effective ingredients, avoiding adverse reactions.

In such cases, your veterinarian may also recommend diagnostic tests to determine exactly what your dog's dietary needs are, such as blood tests or allergy tests.

The importance of supplements

Even with a well-balanced home diet, it can be difficult to provide all essential nutrients solely through food. Supplements such as calcium, omega-3, or specific vitamins may be necessary, but it is essential that they be prescribed by a veterinarian. Improper use of supplements can lead to nutritional imbalances or, in some cases, toxic effects.

Create a partnership with the veterinarian

To get the maximum benefit from veterinary approval, it is important to build a trusting relationship with your veterinarian. Here are some tips for working together effectively:

- **Share detailed information**: Provide your veterinarian with a complete list of the ingredients you plan to use and any recipes you have in mind.
- **Schedule regular checkups**: Monitoring your dog's health status over time is essential for making any

changes to the diet.

- **Be open to suggestions**: Your veterinarian may recommend changes or supplements to the diet based on the latest research or your dog's specific condition.

The role of veterinarians specializing in nutrition

If your general veterinarian does not specialize in nutrition, he or she may refer you to a veterinary nutritionist. These professionals are trained specifically to create tailored diet plans for dogs, taking into account every aspect of their health and needs.

A veterinary nutritionist can:

- **Assess your dog's current diet**: Identify any deficiencies or excesses.
- **Develop a personalized diet plan**: Create recipes that are complete and balanced.
- **Provide ongoing support**: Help you adapt the diet as your dog's needs change.

Dispelling myths about the veterinary approach

Some owners avoid consulting the veterinarian for fear that he will discourage home feeding or insist on commercial foods. It is important to remember that the veterinarian's goal is your dog's well-being. If you choose to prepare food at home, your veterinarian can offer valuable guidance on how to do so safely and effectively.

Veterinary approval is a key step in ensuring that your dog's diet is healthy, balanced, and suited to his needs. Consulting a veterinarian does not mean giving up control of your dog's diet, but working with an expert to offer him the best. With your veterinarian's support, you can confidently approach the home feeding journey, knowing that every morsel your dog consumes is designed to sustain him, nourish him, and make him live a long and happy life.

2. PRACTICES FOR HEALTHY HOME COOKING

THE ESSENTIAL TOOLS FOR COOKING FOR YOUR DOG

Preparing homemade meals for your dog is an act of love that requires attention, planning and the use of the right tools. Just as in the human kitchen, having the right tools and appliances makes the process easier, more efficient and safer. In this section we will explore the essential tools for creating healthy, balanced, and palatable meals for your four-legged friend.

1. Slow cooker: your best ally

The slow stove is one of the most useful tools for cooking for your dog. By cooking slowly and evenly, it preserves the nutrients of ingredients and intensifies natural flavors. It is ideal for preparing stews, soups and complete meals without having to monitor them continuously. Just put all the ingredients in the pot, set the timer and let the slow cooker do the rest.

Why it is useful:

- It saves time and energy.
- Reduces the risk of burning food.
- It is perfect for cooking large quantities and freezing portions for the future.

2. Kitchen scales: for perfect portions

An indispensable tool is an accurate kitchen scale. Cooking for your dog is not just about following your heart, but making sure each meal is balanced. A scale allows you to accurately measure the amounts of protein, carbohydrates, and vegetables, avoiding both excesses and nutritional deficiencies.

What to look for in a kitchen scale:

- Accuracy to the gram.
- Ease of use.
- A wide platform for conveniently weighing various types of foods.

3. Sharp knives and cutting boards

Cutting meat, vegetables and other ingredients requires good quality knives. A well-sharpened knife not only makes the job easier, but is also safer because it reduces the risk of slipping while cutting.

Recommended cutting boards:

- Use separate cutting boards for raw meat and vegetables to prevent cross-contamination.
- Choose materials that are durable and easy to clean, such as plastic or bamboo.

4. Nonstick pots and pans

Nonstick pots and pans are perfect for cooking proteins such as meat and fish without adding excess fat. They also make it easy to clean up, which is important when cooking regularly for your dog.

Helpful hint:

- Use stainless steel cookware or cookware lined with safe materials to avoid chemical contamination.

5. Blender or mixer

To prepare meals that are easier to digest or for older dogs with dental problems, a blender or mixer is an indispensable tool. You can use it to create pureed vegetables, sauces or creamy soups while still ensuring a complete nutritional intake.

Purchase advice:

- Choose a blender with different speeds for more control over consistency.
- Opt for a model that is easy to clean, as you will be preparing fresh meals regularly.

6. Airtight containers

Good storage is essential to keep food fresh and safe. Use airtight containers to store portions prepared in advance, either in the refrigerator or freezer. This helps you organize meals and reduces food waste.

Ideal features:

- BPA-free materials.
- Various sizes to fit different portions.
- Freeze and microwave resistant.

7. Measuring spoons and cups

To follow recipes and make sure your dog gets the right amount of each ingredient, it is essential to have reliable measuring spoons and cups. These tools help you maintain consistency in proportions and follow veterinarian-approved feeding plans.

8. Steamer

Steamers are excellent for cooking vegetables while keeping their nutritional properties intact. As opposed to boiling, which can leach vitamins and minerals into the water, steaming better preserves flavor and nutrients.

Ideal for:

- Spinach, carrots, zucchini and other vegetables safe for dogs.
- Fish or lean meat for gentle cooking.

9. Kitchen thermometer

A kitchen thermometer is a useful tool to ensure that meat and fish are cooked to the right temperature. This reduces the risk of bacterial contamination, such as that caused by Salmonella or E. coli, and ensures safe meals for your dog.

Recommended temperatures:

- Meat: at least 70°C /158°F to eliminate harmful bacteria.
- Fish: around 63°C / 145,5°F for complete but gentle cooking.

10. Grater and peeler

These simple but versatile tools are useful for preparing ingredients such as carrots, potatoes, or zucchini. A grater allows you to reduce vegetables into smaller, easily digestible pieces, while a peeler is perfect for removing unwanted peels.

11. Table of ingredients and meal planner

Although not a physical tool, a meal planner is an essential addition to your cooking routine. A notebook or magnetic board to plan the week's meals will help you save time and ensure a varied and balanced diet for your dog.

What to include:

- List of fresh and dry ingredients.
- Notes on essential nutrients.
- Portion planning according to the dog's needs.

12. Supporting freezer

If you plan to prepare large quantities of food for your dog, a spacious freezer is essential. You can divide the food into daily or weekly portions, making sure they are easy to thaw and serve.

Cooking for your dog may seem like a big responsibility, but with the right tools it becomes a simple, efficient and even fun process. Each utensil or appliance described in this guide is intended to simplify meal preparation and ensure that your dog gets safe, nutritious food. With a well-equipped kitchen and a little organization, you can create homemade meals that will not only meet your dog's needs but also strengthen the special bond you share.

HOW TO SELECT FRESH AND NUTRITIOUS INGREDIENTS

Preparing homemade meals for your dog is a loving way to care for his well-being, but the quality of the ingredients is critical to ensure that the meals are not only delicious, but also healthy and balanced. Choosing fresh, nutritious ingredients is the first step in giving your dog everything he needs to live a long and happy life. In this guide we will explore how to select the best foods, avoiding common mistakes and focusing on options that are safe and beneficial for your four-legged friend.

1. The golden rule: freshness first

The freshness of ingredients is a crucial element in ensuring maximum nutritional intake. Fresh foods not only taste better but also keep intact their essential nutrients, such as vitamins, minerals, and antioxidants, which can deteriorate over time.

How to make sure the ingredients are fresh:

- **Fruits and vegetables**: Look for produce with a bright appearance, without dents or dark spots. Crisp green leaves are a sign of freshness for vegetables such as spinach or lettuce.

- **Meat and fish**: Meat should have a natural color (not too dark or pale) and not give off unpleasant odors. Fresh fish has clear eyes, shiny skin and a mild sea odor.
- **Eggs**: Dip eggs in water; fresh ones sink, while old ones tend to float.

Buy fresh ingredients in small quantities so you can use them quickly without risking spoilage.

2. Meat and protein: choosing the basis for dog health

Protein is the most important component in a dog's diet. Therefore, it is essential to choose high-quality meat and fish that are free of chemical preservatives or artificial additives.

Ideal options for meat:

- **Chicken and turkey**: Lean and easily digestible, they are perfect for most dogs.
- **Beef**: A source of iron and vitamin B12, useful for energy and blood health.
- **Lamb**: Rich in healthy fats, it is a good option for dogs with intolerances to other proteins.
- **Rabbit and duck**: Great for dogs with food sensitivities or allergies.

Recommended fish:

- **Salmon and sardines**: Rich in omega-3s, they support healthy skin, coat and joints.
- **Cod**: Light and easily digested, ideal for dogs with sensitive stomachs.

When buying meat and fish, choose high-quality fresh or frozen cuts, avoiding processed or prepackaged products with sauces and seasonings.

3. Vegetables: a source of essential nutrients

Vegetables are rich in fiber, vitamins and minerals that support your dog's digestion and immune system. However, not all vegetables are safe for dogs, so it is important to be careful.

Safe and nutritious vegetables:

- **Carrots**: Rich in beta-carotene, they are good for the eyes and immune system.
- **Zucchini**: Light and easily digested, they are a good source of fiber.
- **Spinach**: Contains iron, vitamins and antioxidants, but should be offered in moderation.
- **Broccoli**: A powerful antioxidant, but to be served in small amounts to avoid intestinal gas.

Vegetables to avoid:

- Onions, garlic, leeks and shallots: Toxic to dogs.
- Avocado: Contains persin, a potentially dangerous substance.

Buy organic vegetables whenever possible to avoid pesticides and other chemicals.

4. Fruits: sweet natural delicacies.

Fruit is a great addition to your dog's diet, but it should be offered in moderation, as it contains natural sugars. Choose fresh, ripe fruit, removing seeds and stones, which can be toxic.

Safe fruits:

- **Apples**: A good source of fiber and vitamin C, as long as they are seedless.
- **Bananas**: Rich in potassium, but serve in small amounts to avoid glycemic spikes.
- **Blueberries**: Rich in antioxidants, they support brain and heart health.
- **Watermelon**: Moisturizing and low in calories, seedless.

Fruits to avoid:

- Grapes and raisins: Can cause kidney failure.
- Cherries: Pits contain cyanide.

5. Complex carbohydrates: sustainable energy

Although dogs do not need carbohydrates as much as humans, including them in the diet can provide energy and aid digestion. Choose complex carbohydrates, which release energy slowly and are more nutritious.

Recommended carbohydrates:

- **Brown rice**: Easy to digest and rich in fiber.
- **Sweet potatoes**: A source of complex carbohydrates and beta-carotene.
- **Quinoa**: Gluten-free and rich in protein.
- **Oats**: Ideal for dogs with sensitive stomachs.

Avoid refined carbohydrates, such as white bread or pasta, which offer little nutritional value.

6. Oils and fats: support for skin and hair

Healthy oils and fats are essential for maintaining a shiny coat and healthy skin. Include natural sources of omega-3 and omega-6 fatty acids in your dog's diet.

Recommended oils:

- **Fish oil**: Rich in omega-3, ideal for joint health.
- **Flaxseed oil**: A plant-based alternative to omega-3s.
- **Coconut oil**: Supports digestion and skin health.

Use oils in moderation to avoid excessive caloric intake.

7. Quality control of ingredients

The quality of ingredients is crucial to your dog's health. Here are some tips to ensure it:

- **Read labels**: If you buy packaged products, avoid those with artificial ingredients, chemical preservatives or added sugars.
- **Buy locally**: Supporting local markets not only ensures fresh ingredients, but also reduces environmental impact.
- **Freeze leftovers**: If you have excess ingredients, freeze them to keep them fresh longer.

8. Security considerations.

When selecting and preparing ingredients, keep some safety rules in mind:

- **Wash fruits and vegetables thoroughly** to remove pesticide residues.
- **Remove cooked bones from meat**, which can splinter and cause internal damage.
- **Store ingredients properly** to prevent bacterial contamination.

Selecting fresh, nutritious ingredients is the foundation for healthy, balanced home cooking for your dog. With a little care and attention, you can ensure that each meal is rich in flavor and beneficial to his well-being. Investing in quality food not only improves your dog's health, but also strengthens the special bond you share. The time and effort you put into choosing ingredients will be rewarded by the smile (and wagging tail) of your furry friend!

SAFE FOOD PREPARATION AND STORAGE

Cooking for your dog is an act of love that requires attention, care and a safe approach at every stage, from preparation to food storage. Proper handling of ingredients and cooked food not only ensures a healthy meal, but also protects your dog from possible health problems related to contamination, spoilage or nutritional imbalances. In this guide we will explore best practices for safely preparing and storing food for your four-legged friend.

1. Wash and prepare the ingredients

Food safety begins with proper handling of ingredients. Thoroughly washing fruits and vegetables eliminates pesticide residues, bacteria, and dirt, while careful preparation reduces the risks associated with contamination or errors.

Practical advice:

- **Fruits and vegetables**: Use running water to wash each piece. For foods such as spinach or lettuce, soak the leaves in water with a little baking soda, then rinse well.
- **Meat and fish**: Avoid washing them, as the water may spread bacteria to kitchen surfaces. Instead, focus

on cooking them at safe temperatures.

- **Remove toxic parts**: Remove seeds, pits and inedible peels from fruits such as apples and bananas. The leaves of some vegetables, such as potatoes, can also be toxic.

2. Cut and prepare appropriately

The size and cut type of ingredients can affect their digestibility and safety. For smaller dogs or those with dental problems, reducing foods into smaller pieces or creating a soft texture is essential.

Useful tools:

- **Sharp knives**: Reduce the risk of crushing or damaging delicate ingredients.
- **Separate** cutting boards: Use separate cutting boards for raw meat and vegetables to avoid cross-contamination.
- **Blenders or mixers**: Perfect for creating purees or blending hard-to-digest ingredients.

3. Safe Cooking.

Cooking is a crucial step in ensuring food safety. Cooking at proper temperatures eliminates harmful bacteria such as Salmonella or E. coli, protecting your dog from potential infection.

Cooking guidelines:

- **Safe internal temperature**: Use a kitchen thermometer to ensure that meat and fish reach sufficient temperatures:
  - Meat: at least 70°C / 158°F.
  - Fish: at least 63°C / 145,5°F.
- **Cooking Method**: Steaming, boiling, and using a slow cooker are ideal methods for preserving nutrients.
- **Avoid oils and seasonings**: Spices, salt and other seasonings used in human cooking can be harmful to dogs.

4. Cooling and storing food

Once cooked, food must be cooled properly before being stored. Leaving food at room temperature for too long increases the risk of bacterial growth.

Cooling tips:

- **Cool quickly**: After cooking, transfer food to shallow containers to speed up cooling.
- **Do not exceed two hours**: Store food in the refrigerator or freezer within two hours of cooking.

5. Refrigerator and freezer storage

Proper storage is essential to maintain the freshness and safety of prepared food. Use airtight containers to protect food from contamination and oxidation.

Refrigerated storage:

- **Shelf life**: Most dog foods can be stored in the refrigerator for 3-5 days.
- **Transparent containers**: Choose transparent containers to quickly see what each portion contains.

Freezer storage:

- **Shelf life**: Frozen foods can be stored for up to three months.
- **Individual portions**: Freezes food in individual portions to simplify thawing and reduce waste.

6. Thaw Safely

How you thaw food is just as important as how you store it. Thawing improperly can promote the growth of bacteria.

Safe methods of thawing:

- **Refrigerator**: Transfer frozen food to the refrigerator and let it thaw slowly overnight.
- **Microwave**: Use the defrost option for foods that need to be used immediately.
- **Do not thaw at room temperature**: This method can allow bacteria to grow on the outside of the food.

7. Labeling and organization

Properly labeling and organizing stored food is critical to avoid confusion and ensure that food is consumed within safe times.

Advice on labeling:

- **Preparation date**: Write clearly the date you cooked the food.
- **Content**: Specifies main ingredients to facilitate selection.
- **Durability**: Indicates the period within which to consume the product.

8. Preventing contamination

Contamination is one of the greatest risks during food preparation and storage. Follow these practices to ensure safety:

- **Personal hygiene**: Wash hands thoroughly before and after handling ingredients.
- **Clean surfaces**: Disinfect surfaces, utensils and cutting boards regularly.
- **Separate containers**: Stores raw meat, fish and vegetables separately.

9. Safe disposal of waste

Properly managing food waste is important to avoid contamination and maintain a safe environment in the kitchen.

Suggestions for disposal:

- **Get rid of scraps now**: Remove remnants of raw meat, vegetable peels and other potentially harmful residues.
- **Use sealed** bags: Contain waste in sealed bags before disposing of it.
- **Avoid the compost bin for some ingredients**: Bones, raw meat and dairy products should not be composted.

10. Monitor the food prepared

Even with the best storage practices, it is important to check food regularly for spoilage.

Signs of deterioration:

- **Strange odor**: An unpleasant or different than usual odor is a clear sign of deterioration.
- **Abnormal appearance**: Changes in color, mold or texture indicate that the food is no longer safe.
- **Consistency**: Food that appears slimy or sticky should be discarded.

Preparing and storing food for your dog safely is an important responsibility, but with the right practices it can become a simple and rewarding routine. Following these guidelines will help you keep the quality of homemade meals high and protect your four-legged friend's health. The care you put into food preparation and storage will result in a healthier, happier and more energetic life for your dog, who will appreciate every bite knowing it is made with love.

COMMON MISTAKES TO AVOID

Cooking for your dog is an act full of love, but even the best intentions can lead to mistakes that, in the long run, can compromise your four-legged friend's health. Some mistakes may stem from a lack of information, others from the idea that what is healthy for humans is automatically healthy for dogs. To ensure a healthy, balanced and safe home diet, it is important to know and prevent these common mistakes. In this section we will see what they are and how to avoid them.

1. Do not consult the veterinarian

One of the most common mistakes is to start cooking for your dog without first consulting a veterinarian or pet nutritionist. Every dog has specific nutritional needs based on breed, age, lifestyle and any health conditions.

Creating a diet without professional support can lead to nutrient deficiencies or excesses, with potentially serious consequences.

What to do instead:

- Always consult a veterinarian to discuss your dog's nutritional needs before making significant changes to his diet.
- Work with a trained nutritionist to create a balanced, personalized diet plan.

2. Thinking that all human foods are safe for dogs

A common mistake is to believe that human food is automatically dog-friendly. In reality, many foods that are part of our diet can be toxic or harmful to our furry friends.

Foods to absolutely avoid:

- **Chocolate**: Contains theobromine, which is toxic to dogs.
- **Onion and garlic**: They can cause anemia.
- **Grapes and raisins**: Can lead to kidney failure.
- **Avocado**: Contains persin, which can be dangerous to dogs.

What to do instead:

- Inform yourself about safe and dangerous foods for dogs.
- Offer only foods that you know are suitable and prepare meals without adding spices, salt or sugar.

3. Not balancing nutrients properly

Another common mistake is creating unbalanced meals, focusing too much on one type of food (e.g., meat only) and neglecting other essential nutrients such as carbohydrates, fats, and vitamins.

What to do instead:

- Make sure each meal includes:
    - **Protein**: The basis of the dog's diet.
    - **Carbohydrates**: Sustainable energy sources.
    - **Healthy fats**: For healthy skin and hair.
    - **Vegetables**: For vitamins, minerals and fiber.
- Use supplements if necessary, but only on the advice of your veterinarian.

4. Ignoring Safety in Preparation

Cross-contamination and improper food handling can put your dog's health at risk. Bacteria such as Salmonella and Listeria can be found in raw meat and pose a danger if not handled properly.

What to do instead:

- Always wash your hands before and after handling raw meat.
- Use separate cutting boards for meat and vegetables.
- Cook foods at safe temperatures to eliminate any bacteria.

5. Do not monitor portions

A frequent mistake is to offer portions that are too large or too small. Both extremes can cause problems: too much food can lead to obesity, while too little can cause nutritional deficiencies.

What to do instead:

- Calculate your dog's daily caloric needs based on weight, age and activity level.
- Use a kitchen scale to measure quantities accurately.

6. Not storing food properly

Even the best meal can become dangerous if it is not stored properly. Poorly stored foods can develop bacteria or mold, which can be harmful to your dog.

What to do instead:

- It cools cooked food within two hours.
- Use airtight containers to store it in the refrigerator or freezer.
- Check the quality of stored food regularly to prevent it from going bad.

7. Changing the diet too abruptly

A sudden switch from a commercial diet to a homemade one can cause digestive disorders such as diarrhea or vomiting.

What to do instead:

- Introduce the new diet gradually, mixing small amounts of homemade food with the usual food and gradually increasing the amount over a week.

8. Do not monitor the dog's health

Even with the best of intentions, it is easy to overlook small signs that the diet may not be suitable. For example, a dull coat, lethargy, or digestive problems may be signs of nutritional deficiencies or imbalances.

What to do instead:

- Regularly check your dog's health status, including weight, energy and coat appearance.
- Schedule periodic checkups with the veterinarian to evaluate the effectiveness of the diet.

9. Thinking that the home diet is a static process

Your dog's nutritional needs may change over time, depending on age, health, and lifestyle.

What to do instead:

- Re-evaluate your dog's diet regularly with the support of a veterinarian.
- Adjust portions and ingredients to meet new needs.

Avoiding common mistakes in home cooking for your dog is the first step in ensuring a safe and nutritious diet. With a little care and the help of a veterinarian, you can turn every meal into a source of well-being and happiness for your four-legged friend. Remember, your commitment is a valuable gift to your dog, who will appreciate every lovingly prepared bite.

3. START COOKING ON LOW HEAT

WHY THE SLOW COOKER IS PERFECT FOR DOG RECIPES

The slow cooker is a simple but incredibly versatile appliance that can revolutionize the way you prepare food for your dog. This tool, originally designed to simplify the lives of those who cook for the family, has proven equally useful for creating healthy, nutritious and appetizing meals for our four-legged friends. In this chapter, we will explore why the slow stove is an ideal choice for cooking homemade food for dogs, analyzing its practical, nutritional, and logistical benefits.

1. Conservation of nutrients

One of the main advantages of the slow cooker is its ability to preserve the nutrients in ingredients. Slow cooking at a low temperature reduces the degradation of vitamins and minerals that can occur with high-temperature cooking methods such as boiling or frying.

Why it is important for dogs:

- Vegetables keep their essential nutrients, such as B vitamins and vitamin C, intact.
- Animal proteins retain their quality without becoming hard or dry.
- Starches, such as rice or sweet potatoes, soften without losing their energy value.

This means that every meal prepared with the slow cooker is not only tasty, but also packed with nutrients vital to your dog's health.

2. Convenience and time saving

The slow cooker is synonymous with convenience. Once you have prepared the ingredients and set up the machine, you can let it work while you get on with other tasks. This is especially useful for those who have busy lives but still want to provide their dog with home-cooked meals.

Practical benefits:

- You can prepare large quantities of food at one time, freezing portions for later use.
- No need to constantly monitor cooking: just set the timer and let the slow cooker do its thing.
- It is ideal for families who want to cook meals for both humans and dogs, using similar ingredients (but tailoring recipes to each person's needs).

3. Perfect for adapting recipes

The slow cooker is incredibly versatile and allows you to prepare a wide range of recipes. You can combine protein, vegetables, and carbohydrates in one container, simplifying the preparation process.

Examples of dishes suitable for the slow cooker:

- **Meat and vegetable stews**: Chicken with carrots, zucchini and brown rice.
- **Nutritious soups**: Beef broth with sweet potatoes and spinach.
- **Creamy blends**: Lentils with turkey and pumpkin.

The ability to mix ingredients evenly ensures that each bite is balanced and full of flavor.

4. Improved food safety

Slow cooking is ideal to ensure that all ingredients are fully cooked, eliminating any harmful bacteria or parasites. This is especially important for foods of animal origin, such as meat and fish.

How to ensure safety:

- Use a kitchen thermometer to check that the internal temperature reaches at least 70°C / 158°F for meat and 63°C / 145,40°F for fish.
- Be sure to use fresh, quality ingredients that are free of preservatives or chemical additives.

5. Improves digestibility

The slow cooker naturally softens food, making it easier for your dog to chew and digest. This is especially useful for older dogs, puppies or animals with dental problems.

Digestive benefits:

- Starches become more digestible through long cooking.
- The fibers in vegetables break down, making it easier to absorb nutrients.
- The meat softens without losing its protein value.

An easily digestible meal helps prevent gastrointestinal problems and improves the dog's overall well-being.

6. Economical and sustainable

Another reason the slow stove is perfect for cooking for dogs is its economic and environmental impact. You can use less expensive cuts of meat or seasonal ingredients to create delicious and nutritious meals.

Economic benefits:

- Cheaper cuts of meat, such as chicken breast or beef shank, become tender and flavorful through slow cooking.
- You can reduce waste by using parts of vegetables or ingredients that would otherwise be discarded.
- It consumes less energy than a traditional oven or stove that is on for hours.

7. Reduces the stress of preparation

For many owners, cooking for the dog can seem like a stressful endeavor, but the slow cooker makes it easier. There is no need for complex cooking techniques or sophisticated equipment.

Ease of use:

- Just put the ingredients in the slow cooker and set the timer.
- It is not necessary to stir or check frequently.
- Foods can be left to cook overnight or while you are away from home.

This simplicity allows anyone, even beginners, to prepare healthy and tasty meals for their dog.

8. Suitable for special diets

If your dog has special dietary needs, the slow cooker allows you to customize each meal. You can adjust recipes to include or exclude certain ingredients based on your veterinarian's recommendations.

Examples of special diets:

- **Low-fat diets**: Use lean meat and low-calorie vegetables.
- **Hypoallergenic diets**: Choose alternative proteins, such as duck or venison, and allergen-free ingredients.
- **Meals for senior dogs**: Includes easily digestible ingredients and joint supplements, such as fish oil or

flaxseed.

The slow cooker is an indispensable ally for those who wish to provide their dog with healthy, balanced and delicious home-cooked meals without complications. This tool combines convenience, safety and sustainability, making meal preparation an easy and rewarding experience. With its versatility, you can tailor recipes to meet your dog's specific needs, ensuring that every bite is full of love and nutrition. Investing in a slow cooker is not only a benefit to you, but a gift to your four-legged friend's health and happiness.

TIPS FOR GETTING THE MOST OUT OF YOUR SLOW COOKER

The slow cooker is an incredibly versatile and practical tool for those who want to prepare home-cooked meals for their dog. However, to take full advantage of its potential, it is essential to know a few strategies and tricks that can make the difference between an ordinary meal and one that is perfectly balanced, safe and delicious for your four-legged friend. Optimizing the use of your slow cooker requires attention to detail, but once you become familiar with these techniques, cooking will become a natural and effortless process.

The first thing to consider is the choice of ingredients and their order of inclusion in the slow cooker. Always start with those that require longer cooking times, such as meat and starches, and add the more delicate vegetables toward the end. This shrewdness ensures that each item reaches the right degree of cooking without losing essential nutrients. For example, sweet potatoes and brown rice can be put on the bottom, where the heat is highest, while spinach or zucchini can be added during the last hour of cooking.

Another key aspect is the proportion of liquids to other ingredients. The slow cooker retains liquids during cooking, so it is important not to overdo the addition of broth or water. Too much liquid can dilute the flavors and create a texture that is less palatable to your dog. A good rule of thumb is to start with minimal amounts and add liquids only as needed, particularly if you are making stews or soups.

Temperature is a crucial element in making the most of your slow cooker. Although many recipes suggest low or high heat settings, the secret to a perfectly cooked meal lies in slow, even cooking at a low temperature. This mode allows you to preserve nutrients, soften ingredients and achieve well-blended flavors. If you have time, always choose the slower mode-the result will be more nutritious and digestible for your dog.

Advance preparation is another trick that can simplify your work. Cutting and preparing ingredients the night before and storing them in the refrigerator saves you time in the morning. Just transfer everything to the slow cooker and set the timer. This approach is especially useful for those who have busy days but do not want to sacrifice the quality of their dog's meals.

Cleaning your slow cooker immediately after use is a habit that will help keep it in top condition. Food residue left behind for a long time can stick to the walls, making cleaning more difficult and, over time, impairing the appliance's functionality. If you want to make cleaning even easier, you can use disposable bags specifically for slow cookers, which prevent food from sticking and reduce the time it takes to wash the container.

Don't forget to experiment with different combinations of ingredients and textures. The slow cooker is great for mixing flavors and creating unique dishes, so don't be afraid to try new recipes. For example, you can combine proteins such as turkey or salmon with seasonal vegetables and carbohydrates such as quinoa or basmati rice. Whenever you introduce a new ingredient, make sure it is safe and dog-friendly, and monitor for any adverse reactions.

Organization is another key element. Planning meals for the week helps you maximize the use of the slow cooker and ensures a variety of nutrients in your dog's diet. Dedicate a day to batch preparation: cooking large quantities of food at one time allows you to freeze individual portions, ready to thaw and serve on subsequent days. This strategy will not only save you time, but also ensure that your dog gets fresh, balanced meals every day.

Safety is always a priority when cooking for your dog. Use a kitchen thermometer to make sure the meat is cooked to the right temperature, eliminating the risk of bacteria such as Salmonella or E. coli. Also, if you decide to use bones in your dishes, make sure they are well cooked or, better yet, opt for homemade broths with bones removed to avoid dangerous splinters.

Finally, remember that the slow cooker is a tool designed to make your life easier. You don't have to overcomplicate it: a simple recipe with a few high-quality ingredients can be just as nutritious and tasty as a more elaborate one. The real magic of the slow cooker lies in its ability to transform simple ingredients into flavorful and nutritious dishes, making every meal a special moment for your dog.

By following these tips, you can make the most of your slow cooker, turning meal preparation into an enjoyable and stress-free experience. Every bite you offer your dog will be the result of care, attention and love, ensuring your furry friend a healthy and satisfying diet.

HOW TO ADAPT TRADITIONAL RECIPES FOR SLOW COOKER

Adapting traditional recipes for use with the slow cooker is a simple process, but one that requires some special care to get the most out of this extraordinary tool. The slow cooker works at low and constant temperatures, which changes the way ingredients combine and flavors develop compared to traditional cooking methods. This means that some techniques and timing must be modified to ensure that the dish is balanced, nutritious, and perfectly cooked for your dog.

The first step in adapting a traditional recipe is to consider the amount of liquid. In slow cookers, liquids do not evaporate as they do when cooking on stoves or in the oven. This means that you will have to significantly reduce the amount of broth, water, or other liquids specified in the original recipe. Generally, you only need to add enough liquid to partially cover the solid ingredients, since slow cooking will produce additional moisture from the foods themselves. For example, if a traditional chicken stew recipe calls for one cup of broth, in the slow cooker half a cup or less will suffice.

Another important aspect is the way ingredients are cut and arranged in the slow cooker. Since heat is distributed from the bottom, it is essential to place ingredients that take longer to cook, such as meat and starches, on the bottom, while those that take shorter times, such as delicate vegetables, can be placed on top. Cutting ingredients into uniform pieces helps ensure even cooking. For example, carrots and sweet potatoes can be cut into similarly sized cubes, while zucchini, which cooks more quickly, can be added in the last 30 to 60 minutes of cooking time.

Cooking timings are another element that requires attention. Slow cookers generally offer two heat settings: low and high. A dish that would normally take 30 to 40 minutes on the stove might take 4 to 6 hours on high heat or 6 to 8 hours on low heat in the slow cooker. This flexibility allows you to plan meals for your dog without having to constantly monitor cooking. For best results, use the low heat setting, which allows ingredients to cook slowly and develop richer flavors.

Ingredients that require minimal cooking or may lose texture, such as spinach or peas, should be added toward the end of the process. This not only preserves their texture but also retains essential nutrients, preventing them from being destroyed by long exposure to heat. For example, in a recipe for turkey stew with vegetables, you can add spinach in the last 15 minutes of cooking to ensure freshness and nutritional quality.

Spices and seasonings require a different approach in the slow cooker. Although many recipes for humans include salt, pepper and various spices, these are not suitable for your dog. When adapting a traditional recipe, eliminate any ingredients that might be toxic or unsafe for dogs, such as onion, garlic, black pepper, or chili peppers. Alternatively, you can enhance the flavor of the dish with fresh herbs or unsalted chicken broth, again making sure they are safe for your dog.

One aspect that is often underestimated is the final texture of the dish. In slow cookers, foods tend to become softer than in traditional cooking methods. This is especially helpful for older dogs or dogs with dental problems, but may require the addition of ingredients to give consistency. For example, if you are making a stew and want a thicker texture, you can add already cooked brown rice during the last 30 minutes of cooking or lightly mash some sweet potatoes to create a creamy base.

If the traditional recipe includes steps such as browning the meat or roasting the ingredients, you may wonder if they are necessary with the slow cooker. The answer depends on the result you wish to achieve. Although browning is not essential, it can add depth of flavor to the dish. If you have time, you can brown meat or vegetables briefly before putting them in the slow cooker. Otherwise, the dish will still be delicious and nutritious.

A final tip for successfully adapting traditional recipes is to experiment and take notes. Each slow cooker has its own characteristics, and you may need to make a few attempts to perfect liquid proportions, cooking time, and ingredient order. Keep a notebook in which to jot down your observations so you can easily replicate your dog's favorite dishes or make improvements to recipes.

In summary, adapting traditional recipes for the slow cooker is not only simple, it allows you to create customized, balanced, and flavor-packed meals for your dog. By following these steps, you can turn each recipe into a special dining experience that not only meets your four-legged friend's nutritional needs, but makes him happy with every bite.

STEP-BY-STEP GUIDE TO THE FIRST RECIPE

Preparing your first slow cooker recipe for your dog may seem like a feat, but with the right steps and a little planning, you'll realize how simple and satisfying it is. This guide will take you step-by-step through creating a chicken stew with vegetables and brown rice, a balanced, tasty and nutrient-rich recipe for your four-legged friend.

1. Planning

The first step is planning. Before you start, make sure you have all the necessary ingredients and tools. For this recipe you will need:

- **Boneless and skinless chicken**: about 500g / 17,64oz, preferably breast or thigh.
- **Carrots**: two medium-sized ones, cut into rounds.
- **Zucchini**: one large, diced.
- **Brown rice**: 150g / 5,30oz, washed to remove excess starch.
- **Unsalted chicken broth**: 500ml / 0,13gal, homemade or purchased, but free of salt and seasonings.
- **Fresh spinach**: a handful, to be added at the end.
- **Flaxseed oil**: one tablespoon, to enrich the meal with essential fatty acids.

You will also need a slow stove, a sharp knife, a cutting board, and a kitchen scale to measure ingredients accurately.

2. Preparation

Start by preparing the ingredients. Cut the chicken into uniform pieces of about 3-4 cm, so that they cook evenly. Wash the carrots and zucchini thoroughly, then cut them into rounds or cubes. Rinse the brown rice under cold water to remove excess starch-this step will help prevent it from becoming too sticky during cooking.

3. Assembling the Slow Cooker

Place the ingredients in the slow cooker following a specific order to ensure optimal cooking. On the bottom, arrange the chicken, as it takes longer to cook than the other ingredients. On top of the chicken, add the carrots and zucchini. Pour the brown rice as the next layer, then cover everything with the unsalted chicken broth. The broth should cover the ingredients but not exceed them; if necessary, add a little water.

4. Set the Slow Cooker

Set the slow cooker to **low temperature** and a cooking time of 6-8 hours. Slow cooking will allow the ingredients to blend, creating a meal rich in flavor and nutrition. If you have less time, you can opt for the **high-temperature** setting and reduce the time to 4 hours, but the low-temperature mode is always preferable for maximum quality.

5. Check cooking

Halfway through cooking, gently stir the ingredients to make sure the rice absorbs the broth evenly and nothing sticks to the bottom. Check the liquid level and add some if necessary-rice tends to absorb a lot of liquid while cooking.

During the last hour, add fresh spinach on top of the ingredient mix. The spinach will cook quickly with the residual heat, preserving its nutritional properties.

6. Finishing and serving

Once the cooking is complete, turn off the slow cooker and let the food cool for 15-20 minutes. The meal should have a soft but not watery texture, with the ingredients well blended.

Before serving, add a tablespoon of flaxseed oil. This will enrich the dish with essential fatty acids that are beneficial for your dog's skin and coat. Stir well to distribute the oil evenly.

Serve a portion suitable for your dog's size and needs. If you have prepared a larger quantity, divide the food into individual portions and store them in airtight containers. You can refrigerate portions for up to 3 days or freeze them for future use.

7. Cleaning and maintenance

After serving the meal, spend a few minutes cleaning the slow cooker. Remove any food residue and wash the inner container with hot soapy water. If you use slow cooker bags, simply remove them and quickly wash the pot.

8. Monitor the dog's reaction

Watch your dog carefully after the meal. Every dog is unique, and some may require adjustments in recipe or quantity. If you notice that your dog likes the meal and digests it well, this recipe can become a regular staple in his diet. Otherwise, consult your veterinarian to make adjustments based on his specific needs.

By following this step-by-step guide, you can safely prepare your first home-cooked meal with the slow cooker. Not only will your dog enjoy the taste and freshness of the ingredients, but he will also benefit from a balanced and nutritious diet. The slow cooker proves to be an ideal choice for saving time and effort, allowing you to offer your furry friend a meal prepared with love and care. There is no greater satisfaction than seeing your dog wagging his tail happily as he savors a dish made just for him.

4. PROTEIN - THE BASIS OF CANINE HEALTH

RECIPES WITH CHICKEN: CHICKEN STEW WITH VEGETABLES

Chicken is a versatile and highly digestible protein source that is perfect for your dog's diet. In this section, you'll find 20 creative recipes using chicken as the main ingredient, combined with vegetables and other healthy foods to ensure a balanced and tasty meal. Each recipe is structured to be easy to follow and includes suggestions for variations and improvements.

Chicken stew with carrots and zucchini 1.

Ingredients:

- **400g / 14,11oz chicken breast**: Cut it into cubes to ensure even cooking.
- **2 medium carrots**: Peel and cut into rounds about 1 cm thick.
- **1 large zucchini**: Cut it into thin rounds.
- **300ml / 0,08gal unsalted chicken broth**: If possible, use homemade broth.

Preparation:

1. **Preparation of ingredients**: Place the chicken cubes in the bottom of the slow cooker. Arrange the carrots and zucchini on top.
2. **Add the liquid**: Pour in the chicken broth making sure it barely covers the ingredients.

3. **Cooking**: Set the slow cooker to low temperature and cook for 6-8 hours.

4. **Control and stirring**: Stir gently halfway through cooking and add water if necessary.

5. **Finishing and storage**: Serve one portion warm and store the rest in airtight containers for 3 days in the refrigerator or a month in the freezer.

2. Chicken and sweet potatoes

Ingredients:

- **400g / 14,11oz ground chicken**: You can also use ground chicken meat.
- **2 medium sweet potatoes**: Peel and dice.
- **200g / 7,05oz fresh or frozen green beans**: Cut them into small pieces.
- **300ml / 0,08gal of water**

Preparation:

1. **Arrangement of ingredients**: Put the chicken and sweet potatoes in the slow cooker. Add green beans in the last 30 minutes of cooking time.

2. **Baking**: Bake at a low temperature for 6 hours.

3. **Serving**: Lightly mash the potatoes to create a creamier texture.

3. Chicken stew with pumpkin

Ingredients:

- **400g / 14,11oz of ground chicken**
- **300g / 10,58oz pumpkin**: Cut into 1 cm cubes.
- **1 carrot**: Cut into rounds.
- **300ml / 0,08gal of unsalted vegetable broth**

Preparation:

1. **Preparation**: Arrange the chicken and squash in the slow cooker. Add the carrot on top.

2. **Adding the liquid**: Pour in the vegetable broth.

3. **Cooking**: Set the slow cooker to low temperature and cook for 7 hours.

4. Chicken and brown rice with spinach

Ingredients:

- **400g / 14,11oz of chicken breast**
- **50g / 1,76oz brown rice**: Wash it well under running water.
- **1 handful of fresh spinach**

- 300ml / 0,08gal of unsalted chicken broth

Preparation:

1. **Arrangement of ingredients**: Place the chicken and rice in the bottom of the slow cooker. Add spinach in the last 20 minutes of cooking time.

2. **Baking**: Bake for 6 hours.

5. Chicken with green beans and broccoli

Ingredients:

- **400g / 14,11oz of shredded chicken**
- **150g / 5,30oz green beans**: Cut into small pieces.
- **100g /3,53oz broccoli**: Separated into florets.
- **300ml / 0,08gal of chicken broth**

Preparation:

1. **Preparation of ingredients**: Put the chicken and green beans in the bottom of the slow cooker. Add the broccoli toward the end.

2. **Cooking**: Set the slow cooker for 6 hours.

6. Chicken and red lentils

Ingredients:

- **400g / 14,11oz of ground chicken**
- **100g / 3,53oz red lentils**: Wash them thoroughly.
- **1 zucchini**: Cut into cubes.
- **300ml / 0,08gal of vegetable broth**

Preparation:

1. **Preparation of ingredients**: Place the chicken, lentils, and zucchini in the slow cooker.

2. **Adding the liquid**: Pour in the vegetable broth.

3. **Cooking**: Cook for 5 hours at low temperature.

7. Chicken with carrots and apples

Ingredients:

- **400g / 14,11oz of chicken**
- **2 carrots**: Cut into rounds.
- **1 apple**: Peeled and diced.

- 300ml / 0,08gal of unsalted vegetable broth

Preparation:

1. **Preparation**: Place the chicken and carrots in the slow cooker. Add the apple on top.
2. **Baking**: Bake for 6 hours.

8. Chicken with sweet potatoes and spinach

Ingredients:

- **400g / 14,11oz of shredded chicken**
- **200g / 7,05oz sweet potatoes**: Cut into cubes.
- **1 handful of fresh spinach**
- **300ml / 0,08gal of vegetable broth**

Preparation:

1. **Preparation**: Put the chicken and sweet potatoes in the slow cooker. Add spinach toward the end.
2. **Baking**: Bake for 6 hours.

9. Chicken with peas and zucchini

Ingredients:

- **400g / 14,11oz diced chicken breast**: Cut chicken into uniform pieces for even cooking.
- **150g / 5,30oz fresh or frozen peas**
- **1 medium zucchini**: Cut into thin rounds.
- **300ml / 0,08gal of unsalted vegetable broth**

Preparation:

1. **Preparation of ingredients**: Put the chicken in the slow cooker, followed by the peas and zucchini.
2. **Adding the liquid**: Pour in the broth slowly, making sure it barely covers the ingredients.
3. **Cooking**: Set the slow cooker to low temperature and cook for 6-8 hours.
4. **Stir halfway through cooking**: Check that the peas retain their texture and stir gently.

10. Chicken and rice with black cabbage

Ingredients:

- **400g / 14,11oz chicken breast**: Cut into cubes.
- **50g / 1,76oz brown rice**: Washed thoroughly under running water.
- **100g / 3,53oz kale**: Cut into thin strips.

- 300ml / 0,08gal of unsalted chicken broth

Preparation:

1. **Arrangement of ingredients**: Place the chicken and rice in the slow cooker. Add the kale in the last 30 minutes of cooking to preserve the nutrients.

2. **Cooking**: Cook for 6-8 hours at low temperature.

11. Chicken with potatoes and broccoli

Ingredients:

- **400g / 14,11oz of shredded chicken**
- **150g / 5,30oz potatoes**: Peeled and diced.
- **100g / 3,53oz broccoli**: Divided into florets.
- **300ml / 0,08gal of vegetable broth**

Preparation:

1. **Preparation of ingredients**: Put the chicken and potatoes in the slow cooker. Add the broccoli toward the end.

2. **Baking**: Bake at a low temperature for 6 hours.

12. Chicken and squash with spinach

Ingredients:

- **400g / 14,11oz of diced chicken breast**
- **200g / 7,05oz pumpkin**: Cut into cubes.
- **1 handful of fresh spinach**
- **300ml / 0,08gal of chicken broth**

Preparation:

1. **Preparation**: Place the chicken and squash in the slow cooker.

2. **Cooking**: Set slow cooker to low temperature and cook for 7 hours. Add spinach in the last 20 minutes.

13. Chicken with apples and turmeric

Ingredients:

- **400g / 14,11oz chicken breast**: Cut into cubes.
- **1 apple**: Peeled and diced (without seeds).
- **1 teaspoon turmeric**

- **300ml / 0,08gal of vegetable broth**

Preparation:

1. **Preparation of ingredients**: Put the chicken and apple in the slow cooker. Sprinkle with turmeric and add the broth.

2. **Baking**: Bake for 6-7 hours.

14. Chicken with carrots and rice

Ingredients:

- **400g / 14,11oz chicken breast**: Cut into cubes.

- **2 carrots**: Cut into rounds.

- **50g / 1,76oz brown rice**: Washed thoroughly.

- **300ml / 0,08gal of chicken broth**

Preparation:

1. **Preparation of ingredients**: Place the chicken, carrots, and rice in the slow cooker.

2. **Baking**: Bake at a low temperature for 6 hours.

15. Chicken and green lentils

Ingredients:

- **400g / 14,11oz of ground chicken**

- **100g / 3,53oz green lentils**: Washed thoroughly.

- **1 zucchini**: Cut into cubes.

- **300ml / 0,08gal of vegetable broth**

Preparation:

1. **Preparation**: Put the chicken and lentils in the slow cooker. Add the zucchini toward the end.

2. **Baking**: Bake for 6 hours.

16. Chicken with sweet potatoes and apples

Ingredients:

- **400g / 14,11oz chicken breast**: Cut into cubes.

- **200g / 7,05oz sweet potatoes**: Cut into cubes.

- **1 apple**: Peeled and diced.

- **300ml / 0,08gal of vegetable broth**

Preparation:

1. **Arrangement of ingredients**: Place the chicken, sweet potatoes, and apple in the slow cooker.
2. **Baking**: Bake at a low temperature for 6-8 hours.

17. Chicken and quinoa with spinach

Ingredients:

- **400g / 14,11oz of ground chicken**
- **50g / 1,76oz quinoa**: Washed well.
- **1 handful of fresh spinach**
- **300ml / 0,08gal of vegetable broth**

Preparation:

1. **Preparation of ingredients**: Put the chicken and quinoa in the slow cooker. Add spinach in the last 20 minutes.
2. **Baking**: Bake at a low temperature for 5-6 hours.

18. Chicken with zucchini and green beans

Ingredients:

- **400g / 14,11oz chicken breast**: Cut into cubes.
- **150g / 5,30oz zucchini**: Sliced into rounds.
- **100g / 3,53oz green beans**: Cut into small pieces.
- **300ml / 0,08gal of chicken broth**

Preparation:

1. **Preparation of ingredients**: Place all ingredients in the slow cooker.
2. **Baking**: Bake at a low temperature for 6 hours.

19. Chicken with cauliflower and turmeric

Ingredients:

- **400g / 14,11oz of ground chicken**
- **200g / 7,05oz cauliflower**: Cut into pieces.
- **1 teaspoon turmeric**
- **300ml / 0,08gal of vegetable broth**

Preparation:

1. **Preparation**: Put the chicken and cauliflower in the slow cooker.

2. **Baking**: Bake for 6-7 hours.

---

20. Chicken with carrots and spinach

Ingredients:

- **400g / 14,11oz of chicken breast**
- **2 carrots**: Cut into rounds.
- **1 handful of fresh spinach**
- **300ml / 0,08gal of vegetable broth**

Preparation:

1. **Preparation**: Put the chicken and carrots in the slow cooker. Add spinach toward the end.
2. **Cooking**: Cook for 6 hours at low temperature.

With these 20 detailed and balanced recipes, you can vary your dog's meals while ensuring he gets quality nutrients.

RECIPES WITH BEEF: BEEF STEW AND BROWN RICE

Beef is an excellent source of protein for dogs, rich in iron, zinc and B vitamins, which are essential for the overall well-being of your four-legged friend. Beef, when prepared properly, offers delicious flavor and complete nutrition. In this section you will find 20 beef recipes, all easy to make and ideal for ensuring your dog's healthy, balanced diet.

1. Beef stew with brown rice and carrots

Ingredients:

- **400g / 14,11oz cubed** beef: Cut beef into uniform pieces for even cooking. Prefer lean cuts such as rump or butternut.
- **50g / 1,76oz brown rice**: Wash the rice well under running water to remove excess starch, which could make the dish too sticky.
- **2 medium carrots**: Peel the carrots and cut them into rounds about 1 cm thick.
- **300ml /0,08gal unsalted beef broth**: If you do not have ready-made broth, you can make it by boiling beef bones with water and vegetables for at least an hour, without adding salt or seasonings.

Preparation:

1. **Prepare the Slow Cooker**: Make sure the slow cooker is clean and dry. Combine a drizzle of olive oil in the bottom to prevent the ingredients from sticking, although this is not usually necessary with a slow cooker.

2. **Arrangement of ingredients**: Place the beef cubes in the bottom of the slow cooker. Arrange the sliced carrots on top so they are closer to the heat to soften properly. Add the washed rice on top of the other ingredients.

3. **Add the liquid**: Slowly pour the unsalted beef broth into the slow cooker, making sure it barely covers the ingredients. The rice and beef will release additional moisture during cooking.

4. **Set cooking** time: If you have time, select the slow cook (low temperature) option for 6-8 hours. This will allow the flavors to meld and the meat to become tender. If you are in a hurry, use the quick cooking option (high temperature) for 4-5 hours.

5. **Stir halfway through cooking**: After about 3-4 hours, open the lid and stir gently with a wooden spoon. This helps the rice absorb the liquid evenly and prevents the ingredients from sticking to the bottom. Add a small amount of broth or hot water if the liquid seems to have reduced too much.

6. **Check the cooking**: Toward the end of the cooking time, check that the beef is soft and well cooked, the carrots are tender, and the rice has absorbed the right amount of liquid.

7. **Finishing**: When finished cooking, turn off the slow cooker and let the stew rest for 15 to 20 minutes so it cools slightly before serving it to your dog.

8. **Portioning and storage**: Serve a portion that fits your dog's size. Store the rest in airtight containers: can be refrigerated for 3 days or frozen for up to a month. Thaw and reheat before serving.

Suggestions and Variants:

- **For a creamier dish**: Add a diced sweet potato during preparation. When it is cooked, mash it slightly to thicken the sauce.

- **If you want more crunch**: Add a handful of zucchini rounds in the last 30 minutes of cooking. This will maintain their texture and vibrant color.

- **Make the meal special**: Just before serving, enrich the dish with a teaspoon of flaxseed oil to add omega-3s and improve the health of your dog's skin and coat.

2. Beef stew with sweet potatoes and zucchini

Ingredients:

- **400g / 14,11oz cubed** beef: Cut beef into uniform pieces for even cooking.
- **50g / 1,76oz sweet** potatoes: Peel sweet potatoes and cut them into 1-2 cm cubes.
- **1 medium** zucchini: Cut the zucchini into rounds about 1 cm thick.
- **300ml /0,08gal unsalted vegetable broth**: Prepare broth using fresh vegetables without adding salt or seasonings.

Preparation:

1. **Prepare the Slow Cooker**: Make sure the slow cooker is clean and dry.
2. **Arrangement of ingredients**: Place beef on the bottom, sweet potatoes on top, and zucchini on top.
3. **Add the liquid**: Slowly pour in the broth.
4. **Set cooking**: Cook at a low temperature for 6 to 8 hours.
5. **Stir halfway** through cooking: Stir gently to ensure even cooking.
6. **Check the cooking**: Check that the beef is tender and the sweet potatoes soft.
7. **Portioning and storage:** Follow the instructions for portioning and storage.

Suggestions and variations:

- Add a carrot to enrich the taste.
- Just before serving, enrich with coconut oil.

3. Beef with rice and broccoli

Ingredients:

- **400g / 14,11oz of cubed beef**
- **50g / 1,76oz brown rice**: Wash the rice well.
- **200g / 7,05oz broccoli**: Separate the florets and cut them into small pieces.
- **300ml / 0,08gal of unsalted beef broth**

Preparation:

1. **Preparation**: Place the beef, then the rice and broccoli in the slow cooker.
2. **Add the liquid**: Pour in the broth.
3. **Baking**: Bake for 6 to 8 hours.
4. **Stir** and check **cooking**: Stir and check consistency of ingredients.

Suggestions and variations:

- Use quinoa instead of rice for a protein variant.

4. Beef stew with pumpkin and spinach

Ingredients:

- 400g / 14,11oz of cubed beef
- 200g / 7,07oz pumpkin: Cut it into 2-cm cubes.
- 1 handful of fresh spinach
- 300ml /0,08gal of unsalted vegetable broth

Preparation:

1. **Arrangement of ingredients**: Put the beef and squash in the slow cooker. Add spinach in the last 30 minutes.
2. **Set cooking** time: Bake for 6 to 8 hours.

Suggestions and variations:

- Add a diced apple for a sweet touch.

5. Beef with carrots and peas

Ingredients:

- 400g / 14,11oz of cubed beef
- 2 Carrots: Cut them into rounds.
- 100g / 3,53oz frozen peas
- 300ml / 0,08gal of unsalted vegetable broth

Preparation:

1. **Preparation**: Place the beef and carrots in the slow cooker. Add the peas toward the end.
2. **Baking**: Bake for 6 hours.

6. Beef with cauliflower and potatoes

Ingredients:

- 400g / 14,11oz of cubed beef
- 200g / 7,05oz cauliflower: Separate the florets.
- 100g / 3,53oz potatoes: Cut them into cubes.
- 300ml /0,08gal of unsalted beef broth

Preparation:

1. **Preparation**: Put all the ingredients in the slow cooker.
2. **Baking**: Bake for 6 to 8 hours.

Suggestions and variations:

- Add turmeric for an antioxidant touch.

7. Beef and green beans with rice

Ingredients:

- **400g / 14,11oz of cubed beef**
- **50g / 1,76oz of brown rice**
- **200g / 7,05oz green beans**: Cut them into small pieces.
- **300ml / 0,08gal of vegetable broth**

Preparation:

1. **Arrangement of ingredients**: Put the beef, then the rice and finally the green beans.
2. **Cooking:** Cook at a low temperature.

8. Beef with sweet potatoes and apple

Ingredients:

- **400g / 14,11oz of cubed beef**
- **200g / 7,05oz of sweet potatoes**
- **1 apple**: Peeled and diced.
- **300ml / 0,08gal of vegetable broth**

Preparation:

1. **Preparation**: Put beef, potatoes and apple in the slow cooker.
2. **Baking:** Bake for 6 to 8 hours.

9. Beef with rice and mixed vegetables

Ingredients:

- **400g / 14,11oz cubed** beef: Cut the meat into uniform pieces for even cooking.
- **50g / 1,76oz brown rice**: Wash the rice well under running water.
- **150g / 5,30oz mixed vegetables**: Carrots, zucchini and broccoli cut into small pieces.
- **300ml / 0,08gal of unsalted vegetable broth**

Preparation:

1. **Arrangement in Slow Cooker**: Put the beef, followed by the rice and vegetables.
2. **Adding the liquid**: Slowly pour in the broth, lightly covering the ingredients.

3. **Set cooking**: Cook at a low temperature for 6 to 8 hours.

4. **Stir halfway through cooking**: Check that the rice is absorbing the liquid properly.

5. **Check the cooking**: Make sure the vegetables are soft but not too flaky.

6. **Portioning and storage**: Follow standard instructions.

10. Beef with zucchini and turmeric

Ingredients:

- **400g / 14,11oz of cubed beef**
- **200g / 7,05oz zucchini**: Cut them into rounds about 1 cm thick.
- **1 teaspoon turmeric**: For its antioxidant properties.
- **300ml / 0,08gal of unsalted beef broth**

Preparation:

1. **Prepare the ingredients**: Put the beef in the bottom of the slow cooker, then the zucchini.

2. **Add the liquid and** turmeric: Pour in the broth and add turmeric.

3. **Cooking:** Cook for 6-7 hours, stirring once during cooking.

4. **Finishing** touch: Add a teaspoon of flaxseed oil before serving.

11. Beef stew with spinach and potatoes

Ingredients:

- **400g / 14,11oz of cubed beef**
- **200g / 7,05ozpotatoes**: Cut into cubes.
- **1 handful of fresh spinach**
- **300ml / 0,08gal of vegetable broth**

Preparation:

1. **Preparation of ingredients**: Place the beef and potatoes in the slow cooker. Add spinach in the last 30 minutes of cooking time.

2. **Cooking setting**: Cook for 6 hours at low temperature.

3. **Portioning and storage**: As described above.

12. Beef with peas and brown rice

Ingredients:

- **400g / 14,11oz of cubed beef**
- **50g / 1,76oz of brown rice**

- **100g / 3,53oz peas**: Add frozen or fresh peas.
- **300ml / 0,08gal of unsalted beef broth**

Preparation:

1. **Layout**: Put the beef and rice in the slow cooker. Add the peas during the last 30 minutes.
2. **Cooking:** Cook at a low temperature.

13. Beef with broccoli and cauliflower

Ingredients:

- **400g / 14,11oz of cubed beef**
- **100g / 3,53oz broccoli**: Cut into florets.
- **100g / 0,53oz cauliflower**: Cut into pieces.
- **300ml / 0,08gal of vegetable broth**

Preparation:

1. **Preparation**: Place all ingredients in the slow cooker.
2. **Adding the liquid**: Pour in the vegetable broth.
3. **Cooking**: Cook for 6 hours, checking the texture of the vegetables.

14. Beef with sweet potatoes and peas

Ingredients:

- **400g / 14,11oz of cubed beef**
- **150g / 5,30oz sweet potatoes**: Cut into cubes.
- **100g / 3,53oz peas**
- **300ml / 0,08gal of unsalted beef broth**

Preparation:

1. **Preparation**: Put the beef and sweet potatoes in the slow cooker. Add the peas toward the end.
2. **Cooking:** Cook at a low temperature.

15. Beef and quinoa with vegetables

Ingredients:

- **400g / 14,11oz of cubed beef**
- **50g / 1,76oz of quinoa**
- **150g / 5,30oz mixed vegetables**: Spinach, zucchini and carrots.

- 300ml / 0,08gal of vegetable broth

Preparation:

1. **Preparation of ingredients**: Wash the quinoa and chop the vegetables.
2. **Cooking**: Put everything in the slow cooker and cook for 6-7 hours.

16. Beef with kale and potatoes

Ingredients:

- 400g / 14,11oz of cubed beef
- 100g / 3,53oz kale: Cut into pieces.
- 200g / 7,05oz of potatoes
- 300ml / 0,08gal of vegetable broth

Preparation:

1. **Preparation**: Put the beef and potatoes in the slow cooker. Add the kale in the last 30 minutes.
2. **Cooking:** Cook at a low temperature.

17. Beef and green lentils

Ingredients:

- 400g / 14,11oz of cubed beef
- 100g / 3,53oz green lentils: Wash well.
- 1 carrot: Cut into rounds.
- 300ml / 0,08gal of unsalted beef broth

Preparation:

1. **Preparation**: Put all ingredients in the slow cooker.
2. **Baking**: Bake for 6 hours.

18. Beef with zucchini and turmeric

Ingredients:

- 400g / 14,11oz of cubed beef
- 200g / 7,05 of zucchini
- 1 teaspoon turmeric
- 300ml / 0,08gal of vegetable broth

Preparation:

1. **Preparation**: Put everything in the slow cooker.
2. **Cooking:** Cook at a low temperature.

19. Beef with apple and sweet potatoes

Ingredients:

- **400g / 14,11oz of cubed beef**
- **1 apple**: Cut into cubes (without seeds).
- **150g / 5,30oz of sweet potatoes**
- **300ml / 0,08gal of vegetable broth**

Preparation:

1. **Preparation**: Put the beef, apple and sweet potatoes in the slow cooker.
2. **Baking**: Bake for 6 hours.

20. Beef with spinach and quinoa

Ingredients:

- **400g / 14,11oz of cubed beef**
- **50g / 1,76oz of quinoa**
- **1 handful of spinach**
- **300ml / 0,08gal of unsalted beef broth**

Preparation:

1. **Preparation**: Put everything in the slow cooker, adding the spinach in the last 30 minutes.
2. **Baking**: Bake for 6 to 8 hours.

FISH FOR YOUR DOG: COD FILLETS WITH SWEET POTATOES

Fish, such as cod, is a light protein source rich in essential nutrients for your dog's health. It is especially suitable for dogs with food sensitivities or who require a low-fat diet. Recipes using cod can easily be enriched with vegetables and carbohydrates to create balanced and tasty meals. Here are 20 recipes using cod as the main ingredient that are perfect for your four-legged friend's well-being.

1. Cod fillets with sweet potatoes and carrots.

Ingredients:

- **400g / 14,11oz cod fillets**: Cut them into uniform pieces.
- **200g / 7,05oz sweet potatoes**: Peel and dice.

- **1 medium carrot**: Cut into thin rounds.
- **300ml / 0,08gal of unsalted vegetable broth**

Preparation:

1. **Preparation of ingredients**: Place sweet potatoes and carrots in the bottom of the slow cooker. Add the cod fillets on top.
2. **Adding the liquid**: Slowly pour in the vegetable broth.
3. **Baking**: Bake at a low temperature for 4-5 hours.
4. **Check cooking**: Gently stir halfway through cooking and check that the fish is soft and the vegetables well cooked.

2. Cod with zucchini and spinach

Ingredients:

- **400g / 14,11oz cod**: Cut into medium pieces.
- **1 large zucchini**: Cut into rounds.
- **1 handful of fresh spinach**
- **300ml / 0,08gal of water**

Preparation:

1. **Preparation of ingredients**: Arrange the cod, followed by the zucchini. Add spinach in the last 20 minutes of cooking time.
2. **Cooking**: Set the slow cooker to low temperature and cook for 4 hours.

3. Cod stew and brown rice.

Ingredients:

- **400g / 14,11oz of cod fillets**
- **50g / 1,76oz brown rice**: Washed thoroughly.
- **1 medium carrot**: Cut into cubes.
- **300ml / 0,08gal of unsalted fish stock**

Preparation:

1. **Preparation**: Place the rice, carrot, and cod in the slow cooker.
2. **Adding the liquid**: Pour in the broth and cook for 4-5 hours.

4. Cod and broccoli with sweet potatoes

Ingredients:

- **400g / 14,11oz of codfish**
- **150g / 5,30oz broccoli**: Divided into florets.
- **200g / 7,05oz sweet potatoes**: Cut into cubes.
- **300ml / 0,08gal of vegetable broth**

Preparation:

1. **Preparation**: Put the sweet potatoes on the bottom, followed by the broccoli and cod.
2. **Cooking**: Cook for 4-5 hours at low temperature.

5. Cod with green beans and peas

Ingredients:

- **400g / 14,11oz of cod fillets**
- **100g / 3,53oz green beans**: Cut into pieces.
- **100g / 3,53oz fresh or frozen peas**
- **300ml / 0,08gal of water**

Preparation:

1. **Preparation of ingredients**: Place the cod in the bottom of the slow cooker. Add the green beans and peas on top.
2. **Cooking**: Cook at a low temperature for 4 hours.

6. Cod and lentil stew.

Ingredients:

- **400g / 14,11oz of codfish**
- **100g / 3,53oz red lentils**: Wash thoroughly.
- **1 medium zucchini**: Cut into rounds.
- **300ml / 0,08gal of vegetable broth**

Preparation:

1. **Preparation**: Put the lentils and zucchini in the slow cooker. Arrange the cod on top.
2. **Baking**: Bake for 4-5 hours.

7. Cod with potatoes and zucchini

Ingredients:

- **400g / 14,11oz of cod fillets**
- **150g / 5,30oz potatoes**: Cut into cubes.
- **1 medium zucchini**: Rounded.
- **300ml / 0,08gal of vegetable broth**

Preparation:

1. **Preparation of ingredients**: Arrange the potatoes on the bottom, followed by the zucchini and cod.
2. **Cooking**: Cook for 4 hours at low temperature.

8. Cod and rice with carrots

Ingredients:

- **400g / 14,11oz of codfish**
- **50g / 1,76oz of brown rice**
- **2 medium carrots**: Cut into rounds.
- **300ml / 0,08gal fish stock**

Preparation:

1. **Preparation**: Put the rice and carrots in the slow cooker, then add the cod.
2. **Baking**: Bake for 4-5 hours.

9. Cod with pumpkin and spinach

Ingredients:

- **400g / 14,11oz of codfish**
- **200g / 7,05oz pumpkin**: Cut into cubes.
- **1 handful of fresh spinach**
- **300ml / 0,08gal of vegetable broth**

Preparation:

1. **Preparation of ingredients**: Place the squash and cod in the slow cooker. Add spinach toward the end.
2. **Baking**: Bake for 4-5 hours.

10. Cod with cauliflower and sweet potatoes

Ingredients:

- **400g / 14,11oz cod fillets**: Cut into pieces.
- **200g / 7,07oz cauliflower**: Divided into florets.
- **150g / 5,30oz sweet potatoes**: Peeled and diced.
- **300ml 0,08gal of vegetable broth**

Preparation:

1. **Preparation of ingredients**: Arrange the sweet potatoes in the bottom of the slow cooker, followed by the cauliflower and cod.
2. **Adding the liquid**: Pour the broth over the ingredients.
3. **Cooking**: Cook for 4-5 hours at low temperature.

11. Cod and quinoa with zucchini

Ingredients:

- **400g / 14,11oz of cod fillets**
- **50g / 1,76oz quinoa**: Washed thoroughly under running water.
- **1 medium zucchini**: Cut into rounds.
- **300ml / 0,08gal of unsalted vegetable broth**

Preparation:

1. **Preparation of ingredients**: Arrange the quinoa in the bottom of the slow cooker, followed by the zucchini and cod.
2. **Cooking**: Set the slow cooker to low temperature and cook for 4 hours.

12. Cod with apples and carrots

Ingredients:

- **400g / 14,11oz cod**: Cut into medium pieces.
- **1 apple**: Peeled and diced (without seeds).
- **2 carrots**: Cut into rounds.
- **300ml / 0,08gal of vegetable broth**

Preparation:

1. **Preparation of ingredients**: Arrange the carrots on the bottom, followed by the apple and cod.
2. **Cooking**: Cook for 4 hours at low temperature.

13. Cod and broccoli with green lentils

Ingredients:

- **400g / 14,11oz of cod fillets**
- **150g / 5,30oz broccoli**: Divided into florets.
- **100g / 3,53oz green lentils**: Washed thoroughly.
- **300ml / 0,08gal of vegetable broth**

Preparation:

1. **Preparation of ingredients**: Place the lentils and broccoli in the slow cooker, then arrange the cod on top.
2. **Cooking**: Cook at a low temperature for 5 hours.

14. Cod with rice and turmeric

Ingredients:

- **400g / 14,11oz of cod fillets**
- **50g / 1,76oz of brown rice**
- **1 teaspoon turmeric**
- **300ml /0,08gal fish stock**

Preparation:

1. **Preparation of ingredients**: Put the rice and cod in the slow cooker. Sprinkle with turmeric.
2. **Cooking**: Cook for 4-5 hours at low temperature.

15. Cod with potatoes and spinach

Ingredients:

- **400g / 14,11oz of cod fillets**
- **150g / 5,30oz potatoes**: Cut into cubes.
- **1 handful of fresh spinach**
- **300ml / 0,08gal of vegetable broth**

Preparation:

1. **Preparation of ingredients**: Put the potatoes in the slow cooker, then add the cod and spinach in the last 20 minutes.
2. **Cooking**: Set the slow cooker to low temperature for 4-5 hours.

16. Cod stew with zucchini and cauliflower.

Ingredients:

- 400g / 14,11oz of codfish
- 200g / 7,05oz zucchini: Cut into rounds.
- 200g / 7,05oz cauliflower: Divided into florets.
- 300ml / 0,08gal of vegetable broth

Preparation:

1. **Preparation of ingredients**: Arrange the cauliflower and zucchini in the slow cooker, then add the cod.
2. **Baking**: Bake for 4-5 hours.

17. Cod with green beans and sweet potatoes

Ingredients:

- 400g / 14,11oz of cod fillets
- 150g / 5,30oz green beans: Cut into pieces.
- 150g / 5,30oz sweet potatoes: Cut into cubes.
- 300ml / 0,08gal of vegetable broth

Preparation:

1. **Preparation of ingredients**: Arrange the sweet potatoes on the bottom, then the green beans and finally the cod.
2. **Cooking**: Cook at a low temperature for 4 hours.

18. Cod with red lentils and carrots.

Ingredients:

- 400g / 14,11oz of cod fillets
- 100g / 3,53oz red lentils: Wash well.
- 1 large carrot: Cut into rounds.
- 300ml / 0,08gal of vegetable broth

Preparation:

1. **Preparation of ingredients**: Put the lentils and carrot in the slow cooker, then add the cod on top.
2. **Baking**: Bake for 4-5 hours.

19. Cod and broccoli with rice

Ingredients:

- **400g / 14,11oz of codfish**
- **100g / 3,53oz broccoli**: Divided into florets.
- **50g / 1,76oz of brown rice**
- **300ml / 0,08gal of vegetable broth**

Preparation:

1. **Preparation of ingredients**: Put the rice and broccoli on the bottom, then add the cod.
2. **Baking**: Bake for 4-5 hours.

20. Cod with pumpkin and green beans

Ingredients:

- **400g / 14,11oz of codfish**
- **150g / 5,30oz pumpkin**: Cut into cubes.
- **100g / 3,53oz green beans**: Cut into pieces.
- **300ml / 0,08gal of vegetable broth**

Preparation:

1. **Preparation of ingredients**: Arrange the squash and green beans in the slow cooker, followed by the cod.
2. **Baking**: Bake at a low temperature for 4-5 hours.

These 20 recipes offer a variety of nutritious and tasty options for your dog.

5. VEGETABLES - THE SECRET OF BALANCED NUTRITION

SAFE VEGETABLES FOR DOGS: SPINACH, CARROTS, ZUCCHINI

Vegetables are an essential part of a balanced diet, even for our four-legged friends. Although dogs do not have the same fiber and micronutrient requirements as we humans do, introducing safe and nutritious vegetables into their diets can greatly benefit their overall health by improving digestion, immune system and even coat quality. Among the many options available, spinach, carrots and zucchini stand out for their nutritional properties and versatility in cooking. Understanding their nutritional value and how best to use them is essential to providing your dog with a balanced home diet.

Spinach is a green leafy vegetable rich in vitamins and minerals, including vitamin A, vitamin K, iron and antioxidants. These nutrients play a crucial role in supporting eye health, blood clotting and energy metabolism. In addition, spinach contains fiber, which can promote intestinal regularity. However, as with anything, moderation is important. Spinach contains oxalates, which in large amounts can interfere with calcium absorption. For this reason, it is advisable to lightly cook the leaves before adding them to your dog's meals-this simple step reduces the oxalate content and makes the nutrients easier to digest. Spinach can be added to stews or blended to create a creamy base to mix with protein and carbohydrates.

Carrots, on the other hand, are an excellent option for dogs of all sizes. Crunchy, sweet and low in calories, carrots are an excellent source of beta-carotene, a form of vitamin A essential for healthy vision, immune system and skin. Offering raw carrots as a snack is an easy way to help maintain your dog's dental health, as their hard texture helps reduce plaque buildup. However, carrots can also be cooked for extra softness, which is particularly useful for puppies or older dogs with dental problems. An interesting aspect of carrots is their ability to be incorporated into all kinds of recipes-from soups to stews to becoming main ingredients in homemade snacks such as cookies or purees. The natural sweetness of carrots makes them palatable for even the pickiest dogs.

Zucchini is one of the most versatile and safe vegetables to introduce into a dog's diet. Rich in water, fiber and vitamins such as C and K, zucchini are great for hydrating and supporting digestive health. Unlike other vegetables, zucchini are especially light on the stomach, making them ideal for dogs with digestive sensitivities. One of the characteristics that makes them an ideal ingredient is their ability to absorb the flavors of other foods with which they are cooked, enriching the meal without overpowering other flavors. They can be served raw, cut into thin rounds, or steamed or cooked in a pan with a trickle of water. As with carrots, they can be easily mixed with protein or carbohydrates to create balanced meals.

In addition to their individual nutritional value, spinach, carrots, and zucchini can be combined to create highly nutritious recipes. For example, a stew made with chicken, spinach and zucchini is a balanced meal that provides lean protein, vitamins and essential minerals. Similarly, a puree of carrots and zucchini can be used as a base to supplement grains such as brown rice or quinoa. These combinations offer a wide range of flavors and nutrients, satisfying the dog's palate and supporting his overall well-being.

When introducing vegetables into a dog's diet, it is essential to pay attention to preparation. Washing each ingredient thoroughly is an essential first step to remove any pesticides or contaminants. Also, it is important to avoid adding seasonings such as salt, butter or spices, which can be harmful to dogs. Light cooking, such as steaming or boiling, is generally the safest and most effective method of preserving the nutrients of vegetables without compromising their digestibility.

Despite the benefits of spinach, carrots, and zucchini, it is important to remember that vegetables should only be a part of a dog's meal. A balanced diet requires a proper balance of protein, carbohydrates and fat, with vegetables playing a complementary role. Consulting a veterinarian or animal nutritionist is always recommended before making significant changes to your dog's diet, especially if you are dealing with specific dietary needs or pre-existing health conditions.

In addition, it is critical to observe the dog's response to the newly introduced vegetables. Some dogs may be more sensitive than others, showing symptoms such as bloating or diarrhea if they consume too much fiber. In these cases, reducing the amount or choosing vegetables with a lower fiber content can help avoid digestive problems.

In conclusion, spinach, carrots and zucchini are excellent choices for enriching your dog's diet with essential nutrients. Their versatility in cooking and nutritional benefits make them key ingredients in a balanced home diet.

Offering varied meals that include these vegetables will not only improve your dog's health, but also make mealtime an enjoyable and rewarding experience for both of you. With a little creativity and attention, you can turn every meal into an opportunity to strengthen the bond with your furry friend while providing everything he or she needs to live a long and happy life.

RECIPES: VEGETABLE AND LENTIL SOUP

Vegetable and lentil soups are a nutritious, balanced and flavorful option to enrich your dog's diet. Lentils are a plant-based protein source rich in fiber, iron and B vitamins, while vegetables provide a variety of essential nutrients. Preparing these recipes is simple and allows you to combine flavors and benefits in one dish. In this section you will find 20 detailed soup recipes designed to please your dog's palate and ensure his well-being.

1. Lentil and carrot soup

Ingredients:

- **100g / 3,53oz red lentils**: Wash thoroughly.
- **2 medium carrots**: Cut into rounds.
- **200g / 7,05oz sweet potatoes**: Peeled and diced.
- **500ml / 0,13gal unsalted vegetable broth**

Preparation:

1. **Preparation of ingredients**: Place the lentils, carrots, and sweet potatoes in the slow cooker.
2. **Adding the liquid**: Pour in the vegetable broth making sure it completely covers the ingredients.
3. **Cooking**: Set the slow cooker to low temperature and cook for 6 hours.
4. **Stir** and serve: Stir gently before serving. You can mash the vegetables for a creamier texture.

2. Green lentil soup with spinach

Ingredients:

- **100g / 3,53oz green lentils**: Washed.
- **1 handful of fresh spinach**
- **2 medium zucchini**: Cut into rounds.
- **500ml / 0,13gal of unsalted chicken broth**

Preparation:

1. **Arrangement of ingredients**: Place the lentils and zucchini in the slow cooker. Add spinach in the last 30 minutes of cooking time.
2. **Baking**: Bake at a low temperature for 5-6 hours.

3. Vegetable and red lentil soup

Ingredients:

- **100g / 3,53oz of red lentils**
- **1 medium carrot**: Cut into rounds.
- **200g / 7,05oz pumpkin**: Cut into cubes.
- **500ml / 0,13gal vegetable broth**

Preparation:

1. **Preparation**: Put the lentils, carrot and pumpkin in the slow cooker.
2. **Baking**: Bake for 6 hours.

4. Lentil and broccoli soup

Ingredients:

- **100g / 3,53oz green lentils**
- **150g / 5,30oz broccoli**: Divided into florets.
- **200g / 7,05oz potatoes**: Cut into cubes.
- **500ml / 0,13gal of vegetable broth**

Preparation:

1. **Preparation of ingredients**: Arrange the potatoes, lentils, and broccoli in the slow cooker.
2. **Baking**: Bake at a low temperature for 6 hours.

5. Lentil and cauliflower soup

Ingredients:

- **100g / 3,53oz of red lentils**
- **200g / 7,05oz cauliflower**: Divided into florets.
- **2 medium carrots**: Cut into rounds.
- **500ml / 0,13gal of vegetable broth**

Preparation:

1. **Preparation**: Put the lentils, cauliflower and carrots in the slow cooker.
2. **Cooking**: Cook for 5 hours.

6. Lentil soup with zucchini and sweet potatoes.

Ingredients:

- **100g / 3,53oz green lentils**
- **200g / 7,05oz zucchini**: Cut into rounds.
- **200g / 7,05oz sweet potatoes**: Cut into cubes.
- **500ml / 0,13gal vegetable broth**

Preparation:

1. **Preparation of ingredients**: Arrange all ingredients in the slow cooker.
2. **Baking**: Bake at a low temperature for 6 hours.

7. Lentil and kale soup

Ingredients:

- **100g / 3,53oz of red lentils**
- **150g / 5,30oz kale**: Cut into thin strips.
- **1 medium zucchini**: Cut into rounds.
- **500ml / 0,13gal of vegetable broth**

Preparation:

1. **Preparation of ingredients**: Put the lentils and zucchini in the slow cooker. Add the kale toward the end.
2. **Baking**: Bake for 5-6 hours.

8. Lentil soup with spinach and carrots.

Ingredients:

- **100g / 3,53oz green lentils**
- **1 handful of fresh spinach**
- **2 medium carrots**: Cut into rounds.
- **500ml / 0,13gal vegetable broth**

Preparation:

1. **Preparation of ingredients**: Put the carrots and lentils in the slow cooker. Add spinach in the last 30 minutes.
2. **Baking**: Bake for 6 hours.

9. Lentil and potato soup with broccoli

Ingredients:

- **100g / 3,53oz of red lentils**
- **150g / 5,30oz potatoes**: Cut into cubes.
- **100g / 3,53oz broccoli**: Divided into florets.
- **500ml / 0,13gal of vegetable broth**

Preparation:

1. **Preparation**: Place all ingredients in the slow cooker.
2. **Baking**: Bake for 6 hours.

10. Lentil, pumpkin and spinach soup

Ingredients:

- **100g / 3,53oz of red lentils**
- **200g / 7,05oz pumpkin**: Cut into cubes.
- **1 handful of fresh spinach**
- **500ml / 0,13gal of vegetable broth**

Preparation:

1. **Preparation of ingredients**: Arrange the lentils and squash in the slow cooker.
2. **Cooking**: Set slow cooker on low temperature for 6 hours. Add spinach in the last 30 minutes.

11. Green lentil soup with kale and carrots.

Ingredients:

- **100g / 3,53oz green lentils**: Washed thoroughly.
- **150g / 5,30oz kale**: Cut into thin strips.
- **2 medium carrots**: Cut into rounds.
- **500ml / 0,13gal unsalted vegetable broth**

Preparation:

1. **Preparation of ingredients**: Place the carrots and lentils in the bottom of the slow cooker.
2. Adding the kale: Add the kale toward the end of cooking.
3. **Baking**: Bake at a low temperature for 6 hours.

12. Red lentil and zucchini soup

Ingredients:

- **100g / 3,53oz of red lentils**
- **200g / 7,05oz zucchini**: Cut into rounds.
- **1 medium carrot**: Cut into rounds.
- **500ml / 0,13gal vegetable broth**

Preparation:

1. **Preparation of ingredients**: Place the lentils, carrot, and zucchini in the slow cooker.
2. **Cooking**: Cook for 5-6 hours at low temperature.

13. Lentil soup with sweet potatoes and broccoli

Ingredients:

- **100g / 3,53oz green lentils**
- **200g / 7,05oz sweet potatoes**: Cut into cubes.
- **150g / 5,30oz broccoli**: Divided into florets.
- **500ml / 0,13gal vegetable broth**

Preparation:

1. **Preparation of ingredients**: Arrange the sweet potatoes on the bottom, then add the broccoli and lentils.
2. **Baking**: Bake at a low temperature for 6 hours.

14. Lentil and cauliflower soup with potatoes

Ingredients:

- **100g / 3,53oz of red lentils**
- **200g / 7,05oz cauliflower**: Divided into florets.
- **150g / 5,30oz potatoes**: Cut into cubes.
- **500ml / 0,13gal of vegetable broth**

Preparation:

1. **Preparation of ingredients**: Place the lentils, cauliflower, and potatoes in the slow cooker.
2. **Cooking**: Cook for 5 hours.

15. Lentil and pumpkin soup with turmeric

Ingredients:

- **100g / 3,53oz green lentils**
- **200g / 7,05oz pumpkin**: Cut into cubes.
- **1 teaspoon turmeric**
- **500ml / 0,13gal vegetable broth**

Preparation:

1. **Preparation of ingredients**: Arrange the lentils and pumpkin in the slow cooker.
2. **Adding the seasoning**: Sprinkle with turmeric before pouring in the broth.
3. **Baking**: Bake for 6 hours.

16. Green lentil soup with cabbage and carrots.

Ingredients:

- **100g / 3,53oz green lentils**
- **150g / 5,30oz cabbage**: Cut into thin strips.
- **2 medium carrots**: Cut into rounds.
- **500ml / 0,13gal of vegetable broth**

Preparation:

1. **Preparation of ingredients**: Put the carrots and cabbage in the slow cooker, then add the lentils.
2. **Cooking**: Cook for 6 hours at low temperature.

17. Lentil and broccoli soup with spinach

Ingredients:

- **100g / 3,53oz of red lentils**
- **150g / 5,30oz broccoli**: Divided into florets.
- **1 handful of fresh spinach**
- **500ml / 0,13gal of vegetable broth**

Preparation:

1. **Preparation of ingredients**: Place the lentils and broccoli in the slow cooker.
2. **Adding** spinach: Add spinach in the last 30 minutes.
3. **Baking**: Bake for 5-6 hours.

18. Lentil and carrot soup with zucchini

Ingredients:

- **100g / 3,53oz green lentils**
- **2 medium carrots**: Cut into rounds.
- **200g / 7,05oz zucchini**: Cut into rounds.
- **500ml / 0,13gal vegetable broth**

Preparation:

1. **Preparation of Ingredients**: Place the carrots and zucchini in the bottom of the slow cooker, followed by the lentils.
2. **Cooking**: Cook for 6 hours at low temperature.

19. Green lentil soup with sweet potatoes and spinach

Ingredients:

- **100g / 3,53oz green lentils**
- **200g / 7,05oz sweet potatoes**: Cut into cubes.
- **1 handful of fresh spinach**
- **500ml / 0,13gal vegetable broth**

Preparation:

1. **Preparation of ingredients**: Arrange the sweet potatoes on the bottom, followed by the lentils. Add the spinach toward the end.
2. **Baking**: Bake at a low temperature for 6 hours.

20. Lentil and kale soup with pumpkin.

Ingredients:

- **100g / 3,53oz of red lentils**
- **200g / 7,05oz pumpkin**: Cut into cubes.
- **150g / 5,30oz kale**: Cut into thin strips.
- **500ml / 0,13gal vegetable broth**

Preparation:

1. **Preparation of ingredients**: Put the squash and lentils in the slow cooker. Add the kale toward the end of cooking.
2. **Baking**: Bake for 6 hours.

With these 20 recipes, you can offer your dog a variety of nutritious and tasty soups.

HOW TO MAKE VEGETABLES PALATABLE FOR DOGS

Many dogs, just like humans, can be picky about food, and vegetables are no exception. However, including vegetables in your dog's diet is essential to ensure a balanced intake of vitamins, minerals and fiber. Making vegetables palatable is not just a matter of taste, but also how you present and prepare them. With a few tricks, you can turn even the least liked vegetables into a tasty and indispensable part of your four-legged friend's diet.

An effective way to increase the palatability of vegetables is to lightly cook them. Steaming, boiling, or slow cooking in a slow cooker are all good options for making vegetables softer and more digestible without losing too many nutrients. For example, raw carrots, although crisp and fun to chew, may be less palatable than cooked carrots, which develop a natural sweetness during cooking. Cutting them into small pieces and mixing them with other ingredients makes it more difficult for the dog to separate them from the rest of the meal.

Another strategy is to combine vegetables with foods your dog already loves. Mixing cooked spinach with shredded chicken or adding shredded zucchini to a serving of brown rice can mask the flavor of the vegetables and make the whole dish more inviting. For particularly difficult dogs, blending vegetables into a puree is an excellent option. Purees can be mixed with meat, fish, or unsalted broth, creating a uniform consistency that the dog will eat without hesitation.

Texture plays an important role in how dogs perceive food. Some dogs prefer crunchy vegetables, such as raw carrots or cucumber slices, while others find a soft, creamy texture more enjoyable. Experimenting with different textures will help you discover what your dog likes best. For example, you can try serving baked sweet potatoes cut into cubes or reduced to a smooth cream to use as a garnish for the main meal.

The flavor can also be adapted to the dog's preferences. Adding a little unsalted chicken or beef broth when cooking vegetables can enrich their taste and make them more palatable. Healthy oils, such as flaxseed or coconut oil, can be added to vegetables to enhance their flavor and provide additional nutritional benefits. For example, a tablespoon of coconut oil mixed with cooked zucchini or spinach can turn a simple serving of vegetables into an appetizing meal.

Gradual introduction of new vegetables is another key factor for success. If your dog is not used to eating vegetables, start with small amounts mixed with his favorite foods. Gradually increase the proportion of vegetables over time, allowing your dog to adjust to the new flavor and texture. This strategy is especially useful for more intensely flavored vegetables, such as spinach or broccoli.

To make vegetables even more interesting, you can use them as snacks or rewards during training. Pieces of raw carrots, cooked zucchini or seedless apple slices can be offered as a healthy alternative to traditional dog snacks. This not only encourages your dog to consume vegetables, but also reinforces a positive association with their taste. Remember to choose safe vegetables and avoid some, such as onions and garlic, which can be toxic to dogs.

Variety is essential to keep your dog interested in vegetables. Offering the same types of vegetables over and over can lead to boredom and loss of interest. Alternating between carrots, zucchini, spinach, squash, and sweet potatoes keeps meals interesting and ensures that your dog gets a wide range of nutrients. In addition, using seasonal vegetables not only enriches the diet, but is also more economical and sustainable.

Finally, your attitude toward food can influence the dog's behavior. If you eat vegetables in front of your dog and show enthusiasm for their taste, your dog is more likely to be curious and want to taste them. Imitative behavior is one of the most underrated but often effective strategies for introducing new foods into your dog's diet.

In summary, making vegetables palatable for dogs requires creativity, patience and a little experimentation. With the right approach, you can not only improve your dog's diet, but also help him discover new flavors and textures. Vegetables, once accepted, can become a key part of his diet, contributing to his overall health and well-being.

6. COMPLEX CARBOHYDRATES-ENERGY AND VITALITY

BENEFITS OF RICE, POTATOES AND OATS

Complex carbohydrates are an essential source of energy for dogs, providing the fuel needed to support their daily activities and maintain an active lifestyle. Ingredients such as rice, potatoes and oats, when used properly, can enrich your dog's diet with essential nutrients, supporting overall health and vitality. These foods, when integrated in a balanced way, also provide fiber, vitamins, and minerals important for your four-legged friend's digestive and metabolic well-being.

Rice is one of the most common and versatile carbohydrates widely used in dog diets. Easy to digest and low in fat, rice is particularly suitable for dogs with sensitive stomachs or digestive problems. Among the available variants, brown rice stands out for its higher fiber and nutrient content, such as B vitamins and magnesium. These elements help maintain regular digestion and contribute to the health of the nervous and muscular systems. However, white rice, due to its soft texture and superior digestibility, is often preferred for temporary gastrointestinal disorders or light diets.

Rice can easily be combined with lean protein and vegetables to create complete and balanced meals. For example, a dish of boiled white rice with shredded chicken and cooked carrots not only provides energy but also helps calm the dog's stomach. To further enrich the meal, brown rice can be cooked with zucchini or spinach, offering a mix of flavors and textures. It is important to remember to rinse rice well before cooking to remove excess starch and to avoid adding salt or seasonings, which can be harmful to dogs.

Potatoes, including sweet potatoes, are another excellent source of complex carbohydrates, as well as being naturally rich in fiber, vitamins A and C, and minerals such as potassium. Sweet potatoes, in particular, stand out for their beta-carotene content, a powerful antioxidant that supports healthy skin, eyes and immune system. Their natural sweetness also makes them a very palatable food for even the pickiest dogs.

To use sweet potatoes in your dog's diet, simply steam or boil them until soft, then dice or mash them into a puree. This base can be combined with lean proteins such as turkey or fish and cooked vegetables to create a complete meal. White potatoes can also be used in a similar way, but it is important to always remove the skin and make sure they are well cooked, as raw potatoes contain compounds that can be difficult to digest or even toxic.

Oats, although less commonly used, are an extremely nutritious complex carbohydrate that offers numerous benefits for dogs. Rich in soluble fiber, oats support digestive health and help regulate blood sugar levels. It is also a good source of iron, magnesium and B vitamins, which contribute to energy, muscle strength and skin health. Oats are especially useful for dogs with sensitivities to wheat or other common grains because they are naturally gluten-free.

To introduce oats into your dog's diet, you can prepare a simple gruel of cooked oats with unsalted water or broth. This base can be enriched with pieces of apple or banana (no added sugar) for a healthy snack or with protein such as chicken or salmon for a balanced meal. Oats are also a great ingredient for making homemade snacks, such as dog cookies fortified with natural peanut butter or ground flaxseed.

Incorporating complex carbohydrates such as rice, potatoes, and oats into your dog's diet has many benefits, but it is important to keep a few guidelines in mind. First of all, moderation is key. Carbohydrates should make up only part of your dog's diet, since the main energy requirements come from protein and fat. A diet excessively high in carbohydrates can lead to weight gain and associated health problems.

In addition, it is essential to prepare these ingredients properly to ensure that they are safe and easily digested. Thoroughly washing the rice, peeling and fully cooking the potatoes, and cooking the oats to a soft consistency are essential steps to make these foods suitable for dog consumption. Always avoid condiments such as salt, sugar, butter or spices, which can be harmful to your dog's health.

Another important aspect is variety. Alternating between rice, potatoes, and oats, and combining these ingredients with different sources of protein and vegetables, not only keeps the meal interesting for the dog, but also ensures a broader nutrient intake. For example, a meal of brown rice, turkey, and zucchini can be followed by one of sweet potatoes, fish, and spinach, providing a complete nutritional balance.

Finally, observing your dog's response is essential when introducing new carbohydrates into his diet. Every dog is unique, and some may react differently to certain ingredients. If you notice symptoms such as bloating, gas, or changes in stool, you may need to reduce the amount of carbohydrate or try a different option.

In conclusion, rice, potatoes and oats are three outstanding foods that, when used correctly, can provide energy, vitality and nutritional benefits to your dog. With a little care in preparation and combination with other ingredients, these complex carbohydrates can become a valuable part of a balanced home diet, supporting your four-legged friend's overall health and well-being. Experimenting with different recipes and preparation methods will help you discover which combinations are most palatable to your dog, while ensuring that he gets everything he needs for a long and healthy life.

RECIPES: CANINE TURKEY RISOTTO

Turkey is a lean, nutritious protein that is ideal for dogs of all ages and sizes. When combined with rice, an easily digestible carbohydrate, and enhanced with safe vegetables, turkey can become the basis for a delicious and balanced meal. Canine turkey risotto offers a variety of flavors and textures that make it a versatile and popular option. Here are 20 detailed recipes for creating customized risotto for your dog.

1. Turkey and carrot risotto

Ingredients:

- **400g / 14,11oz ground turkey**
- **50g / 1,76oz white rice**: Washed thoroughly.
- **1 medium carrot**: Cut into cubes.
- **300ml / 0,08gal of unsalted chicken broth**

Preparation:

1. **Preparation of ingredients**: Place the turkey, rice, and carrot in the slow cooker.
2. **Adding the liquid**: Pour in the broth making sure it completely covers the ingredients.
3. **Baking**: Bake at a low temperature for 6 hours.

2. Turkey and zucchini risotto

Ingredients:

- **400g / 14,11oz diced turkey**

- **50g / 1,76oz of brown rice**
- **1 medium zucchini**: Cut into rounds.
- **300ml / 0,08gal of unsalted vegetable broth**

Preparation:

1. **Preparation of ingredients**: Place turkey and rice in slow cooker, add zucchini on top.

2. **Baking**: Bake at a low temperature for 6 hours.

3. Turkey risotto with sweet potatoes

Ingredients:

- **300g / 10,58oz ground turkey**
- **50g / 1,76oz of brown rice**
- **150g / 5,30oz sweet potatoes**: Cut into cubes.
- **300ml / 0,08gal of water**

Preparation:

1. **Preparation**: Put the rice, turkey, and sweet potatoes in the slow cooker.

2. **Cooking**: Cook for 5 hours at low temperature.

4. Turkey risotto with spinach

Ingredients:

- **400g / 14,11oz ground turkey**
- **50g / 1,76oz of white rice**
- **1 handful of fresh spinach**
- **300ml / 0,08gal of chicken broth**

Preparation:

1. **Preparation of ingredients**: Put the turkey and rice in the slow cooker. Add spinach in the last 30 minutes.

2. **Baking**: Bake at a low temperature for 6 hours.

5. Turkey risotto with broccoli

Ingredients:

- **400g / 14,11oz diced turkey**
- **50g / 1,76oz of brown rice**

- **100g / 3,53oz broccoli**: Divided into florets.
- **300ml / 0,08gal of vegetable broth**

Preparation:

1. **Preparation**: Arrange the rice and turkey in the slow cooker, add the broccoli toward the end.
2. **Baking**: Bake for 6 hours.

6. Turkey risotto with carrots and zucchini

Ingredients:

- **400g / 14,11oz ground turkey**
- **50g / 1,76oz of white rice**
- **1 medium carrot**: Cut into cubes.
- **1 medium zucchini**: Cut into rounds.
- **300ml / 0,08gal of chicken broth**

Preparation:

1. **Preparation**: Put all ingredients in the slow cooker.
2. **Cooking**: Cook for 6 hours at low temperature.

7. Turkey risotto with kale

Ingredients:

- **400g / 14,11oz ground turkey**
- **50g / 1,76oz of brown rice**
- **100g / 3,53oz kale**: Cut into thin strips.
- **300ml / 0,08gal of vegetable broth**

Preparation:

1. **Preparation of ingredients**: Arrange the turkey and rice on the bottom, add the kale in the last 30 minutes.
2. **Baking**: Bake at a low temperature for 6 hours.

8. Turkey risotto with lentils

Ingredients:

- **300g / 10,58oz ground turkey**
- **50g / 1,76oz of white rice**

- **100g / 3,53oz red lentils**: Wash well.
- **300ml / 0,08gal of vegetable broth**

Preparation:

1. **Preparation**: Put the rice, turkey and lentils in the slow cooker.
2. **Baking**: Bake at a low temperature for 6 hours.

9. Turkey risotto with pumpkin

Ingredients:

- **300g / 10,58oz ground turkey**
- **50g / 1,76oz of brown rice**
- **200g / 7,05oz pumpkin**: Cut into cubes.
- **300ml / 0,08gal of vegetable broth**

Preparation:

1. **Preparation**: Place all ingredients in the slow cooker.
2. **Baking**: Bake at a low temperature for 6 hours.

10. Turkey risotto with potatoes and carrots

Ingredients:

- **400g / 14,11oz diced turkey**
- **50g / 1,76oz of white rice**
- **150g / 5,30oz potatoes**: Cut into cubes.
- **1 medium carrot**: Cut into rounds.
- **300ml / 0,08gal of vegetable broth**

Preparation:

1. **Preparation**: Put the rice, turkey, potatoes and carrot in the slow cooker.
2. **Baking**: Bake at a low temperature for 6 hours.

10. Turkey risotto with cauliflower and zucchini

Ingredients:

- **400g / 14,11oz ground turkey**
- **50g / 1,76oz of white rice**
- **150g / 5,30oz cauliflower**: Divided into florets.

- **1 medium zucchini**: Cut into rounds.
- **300ml / 0,08gal of unsalted vegetable broth**

Preparation:

1. **Preparation of ingredients**: Arrange the turkey and rice in the slow cooker, followed by the cauliflower and zucchini.
2. **Baking**: Bake at a low temperature for 6 hours.

11. Turkey risotto with spinach and broccoli

Ingredients:

- **300g / 10,58oz ground turkey**
- **50g / 1,76oz of brown rice**
- **1 handful of fresh spinach**
- **100g / 3,53oz broccoli**: Divided into florets.
- **300ml / 0,08gal of vegetable broth**

Preparation:

1. **Preparation of ingredients**: Put the turkey and rice on the bottom, followed by the broccoli. Add spinach in the last 30 minutes of cooking time.
2. **Baking**: Bake at a low temperature for 6 hours.

12. Turkey risotto with zucchini and sweet potatoes

Ingredients:

- **400g / 14,11oz diced turkey**
- **50g / 1,76oz of white rice**
- **150g / 5,30oz zucchini**: Cut into rounds.
- **150g / 5,30oz sweet potatoes**: Cut into cubes.
- **300ml / 0,08gal of unsalted chicken broth**

Preparation:

1. **Preparation**: Place all ingredients in the slow cooker.
2. **Baking**: Bake at a low temperature for 6 hours.

13. Turkey risotto with lentils and spinach

Ingredients:

- **300g / 10,58oz ground turkey**
- **50g / 1,76oz of brown rice**
- **100g / 3,53oz red lentils**: Wash thoroughly.
- **1 handful of fresh spinach**
- **300ml / 0,08gal of vegetable broth**

Preparation:

1. **Preparation of ingredients**: Put the rice, turkey and lentils in the slow cooker. Add spinach in the last 30 minutes.
2. **Baking**: Bake at a low temperature for 5-6 hours.

14. Turkey risotto with pumpkin and carrots

Ingredients:

- **400g / 14,11oz ground turkey**
- **50g / 1,76oz of white rice**
- **200g / 7,05oz pumpkin**: Cut into cubes.
- **1 medium carrot**: Cut into rounds.
- **300ml / 0,08gal of vegetable broth**

Preparation:

1. **Preparation of ingredients**: Place the turkey and rice in the slow cooker, followed by the squash and carrot.
2. **Baking**: Bake at a low temperature for 6 hours.

15. Turkey risotto with kale and potatoes

Ingredients:

- **400g / 14,11oz ground turkey**
- **50g / 1,76oz of brown rice**
- **100g / 3,53oz kale**: Cut into thin strips.
- **150g / 5,30oz potatoes**: Cut into cubes.
- **300ml / 0,08gal of chicken broth**

Preparation:

1. **Preparation of ingredients**: Arrange the turkey, rice, and potatoes in the slow cooker. Add the kale toward the end.

2. **Baking**: Bake at a **low temperature** for 6 hours.

16. Turkey risotto with spinach and zucchini

Ingredients:

- **300g / 10,58oz ground turkey**
- **50g / 1,76oz of white rice**
- **1 handful of fresh spinach**
- **1 medium zucchini**: Cut into rounds.
- **300ml / 0,08gal of unsalted vegetable broth**

Preparation:

1. **Preparation**: Place the turkey, rice and zucchini in the slow cooker. Add the spinach in the last 20 minutes.

2. **Baking**: Bake at a low temperature for 6 hours.

17. Turkey risotto with broccoli and sweet potatoes

Ingredients:

- **400g / 14,11oz ground turkey**
- **50g / 1,76oz of brown rice**
- **150g / 5,30oz broccoli**: Divided into florets.
- **150g / 5,30oz sweet potatoes**: Cut into cubes.
- **300ml / 0,08gal of vegetable broth**

Preparation:

1. **Preparation of ingredients**: Place the rice, turkey, broccoli, and sweet potatoes in the slow cooker.

2. **Baking**: Bake at a low temperature for 6 hours.

18. Turkey risotto with zucchini and spinach

Ingredients:

- **400g / 14,11oz diced turkey**
- **50g / 1,76oz of white rice**
- **1 medium zucchini**: Cut into rounds.

- **1 handful of fresh spinach**
- **300ml / 0,08gal of vegetable broth**

Preparation:

1. **Preparation**: Put the rice, turkey and zucchini in the slow cooker. Add the spinach toward the end.
2. **Baking**: Bake at a low temperature for 5-6 hours.

19. Turkey risotto with kale and pumpkin

Ingredients:

- **300g / 10,58oz ground turkey**
- **50g / 1,76oz of brown rice**
- **100g / 3,53oz kale**: Cut into thin strips.
- **200g / 7,05oz pumpkin**: Cut into cubes.
- **300ml / 0,08gal of vegetable broth**

Preparation:

1. **Preparation of ingredients**: Place all ingredients in the slow cooker, adding the kale toward the end.
2. **Baking**: Bake at a low temperature for 6 hours.

20. Turkey risotto with carrots and broccoli

Ingredients:

- **400g / 14,11oz ground turkey**
- **50g / 1,76oz of white rice**
- **1 medium carrot**: Cut into rounds.
- **100g / 3,53oz broccoli**: Divided into florets.
- **300ml / 0,08gal of unsalted chicken broth**

Preparation:

1. **Preparation of ingredients**: Arrange the rice, turkey, carrots, and broccoli in the slow cooker.
2. **Baking**: Bake at a low temperature for 6 hours.

With these 20 recipes, your dog will enjoy nutritious and tasty meals. Each risotto offers a unique combination of fresh, easily digestible ingredients.

TIPS FOR MANAGING CARBOHYDRATE INTAKE

Complex carbohydrates play a vital role in a dog's diet, providing sustainable energy and supporting digestive health. However, properly managing carbohydrate intake is essential to avoid nutritional imbalances and ensure that your four-legged friend maintains optimal fitness. The balance of carbohydrates, protein and fat must be carefully calibrated to your dog's specific needs, considering factors such as age, weight, activity level and overall health.

A first step in managing carbohydrate intake in your dog's diet is to determine the type of carbohydrates to use. Complex carbohydrates such as brown rice, sweet potatoes, and oats are preferable to simple carbohydrates because they release energy more slowly, keeping blood sugar levels stable. Brown rice, for example, is rich in fiber and essential nutrients that support healthy digestion and provide lasting energy. Sweet potatoes, with their high beta-carotene content, are an excellent choice for adding vitamins and minerals to your dog's diet, while oats offer soluble fiber that improves intestinal health.

To avoid excessive carbohydrate intake, it is important to adhere to the recommended proportions within the meal. Generally, carbohydrates should constitute about 10-15% of the total daily calories for most healthy dogs. In more active or growing dogs, this percentage may be slightly higher, while in sedentary or overweight dogs, it may be appropriate to reduce it. To achieve an optimal balance, combine carbohydrates with lean protein such as chicken, turkey or fish and healthy fats such as flaxseed oil or coconut oil.

Another crucial aspect of managing carbohydrate intake is to monitor the quality and preparation of ingredients. Brown rice should be washed thoroughly to remove excess starch and cooked to a soft consistency, making it more digestible for the dog. Sweet potatoes should be peeled, steamed or boiled until tender, while oats should be cooked with unsalted water or broth to create a nutritious and easily chewy base. Always avoid adding salt, butter or sugar, which can be harmful to your dog's health.

Observing portion sizes is another essential component of effective carbohydrate management. Although complex carbohydrates are beneficial, too much can lead to weight gain or digestive problems. Start with small amounts, monitoring how your dog reacts. For example, if you notice that your dog is showing signs of fatigue or unexplained weight gain, it may be helpful to slightly reduce the amount of carbohydrates in his meal and increase protein to compensate.

Also, consider alternating different carbohydrate sources to vary your dog's diet and provide a broad spectrum of nutrients. For example, one meal might include brown rice combined with turkey and zucchini, while another might be sweet potatoes with chicken and spinach. Alternating between oats and rice, or sweet potatoes and squash, keeps meals interesting and prevents monotony while ensuring that your dog receives a well-balanced diet.

One aspect often overlooked is the role of the dog's activity level in determining carbohydrate intake. Dogs that engage in regular or intense physical activity, such as running or prolonged play, require more carbohydrate to sustain their energy levels. Conversely, less active or older dogs might benefit from a lower carbohydrate diet to avoid unnecessary calorie accumulation.

Finally, it is critical to consider any specific health conditions your dog may have. For example, dogs with diabetes or glycemic sensitivities may require more stringent management of carbohydrate intake. In these cases, your veterinarian might recommend low-glycemic-index carbohydrates, such as sweet potatoes or oats, and carefully monitor portion sizes and meal frequency.

In summary, managing carbohydrate intake in your dog's diet requires a careful and individualized approach. Choosing high-quality ingredients, adhering to recommended proportions, alternating carbohydrate sources, and considering your dog's activity level and specific needs are key steps to ensuring a balanced diet. With a little care and planning, you can use complex carbohydrates to provide your dog with the energy and vitality needed for a long and healthy life.

7. SUPERFOODS FOR DOGS - POWERFUL ADDITIONS

THE BENEFITS OF FLAXSEED, TURMERIC AND FISH OIL

Superfoods are an outstanding addition to your dog's diet, providing essential nutrients that improve overall health and support specific aspects of wellness, such as the skin, joints, and immune system. Flaxseed, turmeric, and fish oil are three examples of superfoods that can make a big difference in your four-legged friend's life. When used correctly, these ingredients not only enrich your dog's meals, but can also help prevent and manage some common health conditions.

Flaxseeds are an excellent source of omega-3 fatty acids, which support healthy skin and coat, as well as promote good heart function. They also contain lignans, plant compounds with antioxidant and anti-inflammatory properties, which can help reduce chronic inflammation and improve your dog's overall health. To ensure that flaxseeds are easily digestible, it is important to grind them before adding them to the meal. In fact, whole seeds can pass through the digestive tract without being fully absorbed. Once ground, they can be sprinkled on food or mixed into a vegetable puree to enrich meals. The ideal amount varies according to the dog's weight, but generally one teaspoon per day for medium-sized dogs is sufficient to provide the desired benefits.

Turmeric, known primarily as a culinary spice, is also a powerful natural antioxidant and anti-inflammatory. It contains curcumin, a bioactive compound that can help reduce inflammation, relieve joint pain and support liver health. Turmeric is especially useful for older dogs or those with joint problems, such as arthritis. However, to be effective, curcumin needs to be combined with a small amount of black pepper, which increases its bioavailability, and healthy fats, such as coconut or fish oil. A golden paste, prepared by mixing turmeric, black pepper and water until it forms a creamy consistency, can be added to meals in small amounts. Again, the dose varies according to the size of the dog: start with a teaspoon tip for small dogs and gradually increase for larger dogs.

Fish oil is another outstanding addition to your dog's diet because of its high content of omega-3 fatty acids, particularly EPA and DHA. These nutrients are critical for brain, joint and skin health, as well as supporting the immune system. Fish oil can also help reduce inflammation levels and improve mobility in dogs with arthritis. When choosing a fish oil, it is important to opt for one of high quality, preferably purified to remove any toxins or heavy metals. Salmon, anchovy or sardine oils are often considered among the best. You can add a few drops of fish oil directly onto your dog's food, starting with a small amount and gradually increasing to avoid gastrointestinal upset.

When incorporating these superfoods into your dog's diet, it is essential to do so gradually and monitor his reaction. Even natural, healthy foods can cause problems if given in excessive doses or if your dog has special allergies or sensitivities. Always start with small amounts, observing any changes in your dog's behavior, energy or digestion.

One creative way to introduce flaxseed, turmeric, and fish oil is to include them in specific home recipes. For example, you can make a puree of carrots and sweet potatoes with a pinch of turmeric and a splash of fish oil, or add ground flaxseed to a chicken and rice stew. These ingredients not only improve the nutritional profile of the meal, but also enrich the flavor, making it more palatable for your dog.

Another advantage of these superfoods is their versatility. Flaxseeds can also be used as a natural binder to make homemade snacks, such as gluten-free dog cookies. Turmeric can be mixed with natural yogurt to create a creamy and beneficial condiment, while fish oil can be drizzled over any meal for a quick and nutritious addition.

In addition to their physical benefits, these superfoods can contribute to your dog's mental well-being. The omega-3 fatty acids found in flaxseed and fish oil, for example, have been associated with improved cognitive function, making them especially useful for older dogs. Turmeric, due to its antioxidant properties, can help protect body and brain cells from oxidative damage, supporting your furry friend's longevity and quality of life.

An important aspect to keep in mind is that the effectiveness of these superfoods also depends on their storage and handling. Ground flaxseed, for example, should be stored in an airtight container in the refrigerator to preserve freshness and prevent oxidation. Fish oil should also be stored in a cool, dry place away from direct light to prevent it from going rancid. Turmeric, on the other hand, should be purchased in small quantities and stored in a tightly sealed jar away from moisture.

In conclusion, flaxseed, turmeric, and fish oil are three powerful and versatile additions that can significantly improve your dog's diet. With a little creativity and care, you can incorporate these superfoods in a safe and beneficial way, helping your four-legged friend live a long, healthy and happy life.

RECIPES: BLUEBERRY AND CHIA SEED PORRIDGE

Porridge is a versatile and nutritious meal, perfect for including superfoods such as blueberries and chia seeds in your dog's diet. Blueberries, rich in antioxidants, vitamins, and fiber, are great for supporting the immune system and eye health, while chia seeds offer an extraordinary amount of omega-3 fatty acids, calcium, and protein. When combined in a porridge, these ingredients create a balanced, flavorful meal that is easy to prepare and customize to meet your four-legged friend's specific needs. Here are 20 detailed recipes for making delicious and healthy porridge for your dog.

1. Classic blueberry and chia seed porridge

Ingredients:

- **50g / 1,76oz oats:** Cooked with water or unsalted vegetable broth.
- **1 tablespoon of chia seeds**
- **30g / 1,06oz fresh or frozen blueberries**

Preparation:

1. **Preparation of oats:** Cook oats until soft.
2. **Adding ingredients:** Stir the chia seeds and blueberries into the hot oats.
3. **Cooling and serving:** Let the porridge cool before offering it to your dog.

2. Porridge with banana and chia seeds

Ingredients:

- **50g / 1,76oz of oats**
- **1 tablespoon of chia seeds**
- **1 ripe banana:** Mashed.

Preparation:

1. **Preparation of oats:** Cook oats as described above.
2. **Stirring:** Add the chia seeds and mashed banana to the hot oats.

3. Porridge with apple and cinnamon

Ingredients:

- 50g / 1,76oz of oats
- 1 tablespoon of chia seeds
- **1 apple**: Grated and seedless.
- 1 pinch of cinnamon

Preparation:

1. **Preparation of oats**: Cook the oats.
2. **Adding the apple and cinnamon**: Stir the grated apple and cinnamon into the hot oats along with the chia seeds.

4. Blueberry porridge and yogurt

Ingredients:

- 50g / 1,76oz of oats
- 1 tablespoon of chia seeds
- 30g / 1,06oz of fresh blueberries
- 1 tablespoon sugar-free natural yogurt

Preparation:

1. **Preparation of oats**: Cook the oats and let them cool.
2. **Stirring**: Add the blueberries, chia seeds and yogurt.

5. Porridge with pumpkin and chia seeds

Ingredients:

- 50g / 1,76oz of oats
- 1 tablespoon of chia seeds
- 50g / 1,76oz cooked and mashed pumpkin

Preparation:

1. **Preparation of oats**: Cook the oats.
2. **Adding the pumpkin**: Stir the pumpkin and chia seeds into the hot oats.

6. Blueberry porridge and coconut oil.

Ingredients:

- 50g / 1,76oz of oats
- 1 tablespoon of chia seeds
- 30g / 1,06oz of fresh blueberries
- 1 teaspoon coconut oil

Preparation:

1. **Preparation of oats**: Cook the oats.
2. **Blending**: Add the coconut oil, blueberries and chia seeds.

7. Porridge with carrots and chia seeds

Ingredients:

- 50g / 1,76oz of oats
- 1 tablespoon of chia seeds
- 50g / 1,76oz grated carrots

Preparation:

1. **Preparation of oats**: Cook the oats.
2. **Adding the carrots**: Stir the carrots and chia seeds into the hot oats.

8. Blueberry porridge with chopped almonds.

Ingredients:

- 50g / 1,76oz of oats
- 1 tablespoon of chia seeds
- 30g / 1,06oz of blueberries
- 1 teaspoon ground almonds (unsalted and unsweetened)

Preparation:

1. **Preparation of oats**: Cook the oats.
2. **Mixing**: Add the blueberries, almonds and chia seeds.

9. Porridge with spinach and chia seeds

Ingredients:

- 50g / 1,76oz of oats

- 1 tablespoon of chia seeds
- 30g / 1,06oz cooked and chopped spinach

Preparation:

1. **Preparation of oats**: Cook the oats.
2. **Stirring**: Add spinach and chia seeds.

10. Porridge with pumpkin and blueberries

Ingredients:

- 50g / 1,76oz of oats
- 1 tablespoon of chia seeds
- 50g / 1,76oz cooked and mashed pumpkin
- 30g / 1,06oz of blueberries

Preparation:

1. **Preparation of oats**: Cook the oats.
2. **Adding ingredients**: Stir in the pumpkin, blueberries and chia seeds.

11. Porridge with natural yogurt, honey and chia seeds

Ingredients:

- **50g / 1,76oz oats**: Cooked in unsalted water or broth.
- 1 tablespoon of chia seeds
- 1 teaspoon of natural honey
- 1 tablespoon sugar-free natural yogurt

Preparation:

1. **Preparing the** oats: Cook the oats until they have a creamy consistency.
2. **Adding ingredients**: Stir the chia seeds, honey and yogurt into the hot oats.
3. **Chilling**: Let cool before serving.

12. Porridge with apple, cinnamon and chia seeds.

Ingredients:

- 50g / 1,76oz of oats
- 1 tablespoon of chia seeds
- **1 medium apple**: Grated or diced, seedless.

- 1 pinch of cinnamon

Preparation:

1. **Preparation of oats**: Cook oats as described above.

2. **Stirring**: Add the apple, chia seeds and cinnamon to the hot oats.

13. Porridge with sweet potatoes and chia seeds

Ingredients:

- 50g / 1,76oz of oats
- 1 tablespoon of chia seeds
- 50g / 1,76oz cooked and mashed sweet potatoes

Preparation:

1. **Preparation of oats**: Cook the oats and let them cool.

2. **Adding** the sweet potatoes: Stir the sweet potatoes and chia seeds into the oats.

14. Porridge with turmeric and blueberries

Ingredients:

- 50g / 1,76oz of oats
- 1 tablespoon of chia seeds
- 30g / 1,06oz of fresh blueberries
- 1 pinch of turmeric

Preparation:

1. **Preparation of oats**: Cook the oats.

2. **Stirring**: Add the blueberries, chia seeds and turmeric to the hot oats.

15. Porridge with flaxseed, chia seeds and blueberries

Ingredients:

- 50g / 1,76oz of oats
- 1 tablespoon of chia seeds
- 1 tablespoon ground flaxseed
- 30g / 1,06oz of blueberries

Preparation:

1. **Preparation of oats**: Cook oats until soft.

2. **Adding the ingredients**: Stir flax seeds, chia seeds and blueberries into the oats.

16. Porridge with peach and chia seeds

Ingredients:

- **50g / 1,76oz of oats**
- **1 tablespoon of chia seeds**
- **1 medium peach**: Peeled and diced.

Preparation:

1. **Preparation of oats**: Cook the oats and let them cool slightly.
2. **Adding the peach**: Stir the peach cubes and chia seeds into the oats.

17. Porridge with banana, carrots and chia seeds.

Ingredients:

- **50g / 1,76oz of oats**
- **1 tablespoon of chia seeds**
- **1 ripe banana**: Mashed.
- **30g / 1,06oz grated carrots**

Preparation:

1. **Preparation of oats**: Cook the oats.
2. **Mixing**: Add the banana, carrots and chia seeds.

18. Porridge with yogurt and chopped strawberries

Ingredients:

- **50g / 1,76oz of oats**
- **1 tablespoon of chia seeds**
- **2 medium strawberries**: Finely chopped.
- **1 tablespoon of natural yogurt**

Preparation:

1. **Preparation of oats**: Cook oats until soft.
2. **Adding ingredients**: Mix the strawberries, yogurt and chia seeds.

19. Porridge with avocado and chia seeds.

Ingredients:

- **50g / 1,76oz of oats**
- **1 tablespoon of chia seeds**
- **30g / 1,06oz ripe avocado**: Mashed.

Preparation:

1. **Preparation of oats**: Cook the oats and let them cool.
2. **Adding the avocado**: Stir the avocado and chia seeds into the oats.

---

20. Porridge with natural peanut butter and chia seeds.

Ingredients:

- **50g / 1,76oz of oats**
- **1 tablespoon of chia seeds**
- **1 teaspoon of natural peanut butter**

Preparation:

1. **Preparation of oats**: Cook oats as described.
2. **Mixing**: Add the peanut butter and chia seeds.

These 20 oatmeal recipes offer a wide variety of options to enrich your dog's diet with beneficial nutrients and delicious flavors. Each combination is designed to be easy to prepare and adaptable to your furry friend's preferences.

HOW TO INCORPORATE SUPERFOODS INTO DAILY RECIPES

Incorporating superfoods into your dog's diet is an excellent way to enrich his diet and support his overall well-being. Superfoods, such as flaxseed, turmeric, fish oil, blueberries, pumpkin, and many others, are rich in essential nutrients and offer specific health benefits for your dog. However, the addition of these ingredients must be done carefully to ensure that they are well tolerated and suited to your four-legged friend's individual needs. Let's find out how you can easily incorporate superfoods into daily recipes to provide healthy and delicious meals.

Incorporating Flaxseed into Recipes

Flaxseeds are a versatile and nutritious addition due to their high content of omega-3 fatty acids and fiber. To ensure that your dog best absorbs the benefits, flaxseeds should be ground before use. Once ground, they can be mixed with other ingredients or used as a topping.

For example, you can add a teaspoon of ground flaxseeds to a serving of brown rice with chicken and zucchini. Alternatively, you can mix them into a puree of sweet potatoes and spinach, creating a creamy texture that is easy to consume. Flaxseed can also be used to make homemade snacks, such as dog cookies, by replacing some of the flour with ground flaxseed for a nutritional boost.

Using Turmeric for Anti-Inflammatory Benefits

Turmeric, with its antioxidant and anti-inflammatory properties, is ideal for dogs with joint problems or in need of support for general health. To improve its absorption, turmeric should be combined with a healthy fat, such as coconut oil, and a pinch of black pepper.

A simple daily recipe might include a teaspoon of turmeric mixed with coconut oil and added to a turkey, rice and vegetable stew. You can also make a "golden paste" by mixing turmeric and water to a creamy consistency. This paste can be stored in the refrigerator and added to meals in small amounts, fitting perfectly into different diets.

Integrating Fish Oil into Meals

Fish oil is a primary source of omega-3s, which support healthy skin, coat, and joints, as well as promote brain function. This ingredient is incredibly easy to incorporate into daily meals. Just add a few drops of fish oil to an already prepared dish, such as a turkey risotto with spinach, to enrich it with nutrients.

If your dog does not like the smell of fish oil, you can mix it with other more aromatic ingredients, such as carrot puree or pumpkin. In addition, fish oil can be used as a topping for homemade snacks such as salty dog cookies, improving their nutritional value.

Include Blueberries for an Antioxidant Boost

Blueberries, rich in antioxidants and vitamins, are a perfect superfood for keeping your dog's immune system strong and healthy. They can be added to many daily recipes, either fresh or lightly cooked.

For example, you can mix a handful of blueberries into a bowl of cooked oats and chia seeds, creating a nutrient-rich porridge. Blueberries can also be added to a chicken and sweet potato casserole, lending a touch of natural sweetness to the meal.

Using Pumpkin as a Nutritional Base

Pumpkin is a versatile, fiber-rich ingredient perfect for supporting your dog's digestion. It can be easily incorporated into daily meals in puree form or as a main ingredient in more elaborate recipes.

A winning combination might include pumpkin puree, shredded turkey and brown rice. Pumpkin puree can also be used as a base for soft snacks, mixing it with whole wheat flour and a pinch of turmeric to create nutritious cookies.

Add Chia Seeds for Energy and Vitality

Chia seeds are one of the richest plant sources of omega-3, protein and fiber. They can be added to daily recipes to improve your dog's coat and skin health, as well as provide an energy boost.

A simple idea is to mix a teaspoon of chia seeds with natural yogurt and blueberries to create a nutritious breakfast for your dog. Chia seeds can also be added to stews or risottos, increasing the fiber content without altering the flavor too much.

Creating Versatile Superfood Combinations

One of the most effective strategies for incorporating superfoods into daily recipes is to combine multiple ingredients in one meal. For example, a stew of chicken, sweet potatoes, and spinach can be enhanced with a splash of fish oil, a teaspoon of flaxseed, and a pinch of turmeric. This type of recipe not only provides a broad spectrum of nutrients, but is also incredibly tasty and satisfying for your dog.

Experimenting with Homemade Snacks

Homemade snacks are a great way to incorporate superfoods into your dog's diet. For example, you can make cookies by mixing whole wheat flour, pumpkin puree, flaxseed, and a pinch of turmeric. These snacks are not only healthy, but also offer a yummy option to reward your dog during training or as an occasional snack.

Observe Your Dog's Reaction

When integrating new ingredients into your dog's diet, it is important to do so gradually and monitor his reaction. Some superfoods, if consumed in excessive amounts, can cause gastrointestinal upset or allergies. Always start with small amounts and observe any changes in your dog's behavior, digestion or energy.

In conclusion, superfoods such as flaxseed, turmeric, fish oil, blueberries, pumpkin, and chia seeds offer a world of possibilities for improving your dog's diet. With a little creativity and care, you can incorporate these ingredients in a safe and beneficial way, ensuring your four-legged friend a long, healthy and happy life.

8. SPECIAL DIETS AND HEALTH CONDITIONS

FOODS FOR DOGS WITH ALLERGIES OR INTOLERANCES

Food allergies and intolerances are a common challenge for many dog owners. These conditions, which can manifest in a variety of ways, require an individualized dietary approach to improve a dog's health and well-being. We delve into every aspect of diets for dogs with allergies or intolerances, providing details on ingredients, preparation strategies, and practical solutions to address these issues.

Identify allergies and adopt an exclusive diet

The process of identifying food allergies requires patience and observation. Allergies can arise from common proteins such as chicken, beef, or eggs, but also from carbohydrates such as wheat or corn. An elimination diet is the most effective method of isolating allergens: it consists of feeding the dog one source of protein and one source of carbohydrates it has not consumed before, such as fish and sweet potatoes. This regimen is maintained for about 8-12 weeks, during which any improvement in symptoms is closely monitored.

If symptoms disappear, other ingredients can be reintroduced one at a time, with intervals of 7-10 days, to identify those causing adverse reactions. During this period, it is essential to maintain a strict diet and not offer snacks or table scraps, which could compromise the outcome.

Choose alternative proteins and carbohydrates

When selecting ingredients for a dog with allergies, it is important to opt for less common protein and carbohydrate sources that reduce the risk of reactions. Proteins such as lamb, venison, duck or fish are good alternatives to more traditional proteins. Hydrolyzed proteins, found in some veterinary diets, can also be a safe option, as the protein molecules are fragmented so as not to trigger an immune response.

For carbohydrates, sweet potatoes, brown rice, quinoa, and tapioca are excellent choices. These ingredients provide energy and fiber without irritating the dog's digestive system. Preparation is key: fully cooking carbohydrates makes them more digestible and reduces the risk of gastrointestinal upset.

Practical example: a simple but balanced recipe might include 150g / 5,30oz steamed turkey, 100g / 3,53oz boiled sweet potatoes and 50g / 1,76oz cooked zucchini, with a teaspoon of flaxseed oil added to provide essential fatty acids.

Avoid additives and processed ingredients

Industrial dog foods often contain preservatives, dyes and artificial flavors, which can trigger allergies or intolerances. Preparing homemade meals is a safe way to eliminate these substances and fully control the quality of ingredients. It is important to choose fresh meat, organic vegetables and whole-grain carbohydrates. The water used for cooking should also be free of chlorine or contaminants, as these can adversely affect some sensitive dogs.

An additional advantage of homemade meals is the ability to tailor portions and ingredients to the specific needs of the dog, ensuring that the diet is not only safe but also nutritionally balanced.

Include beneficial superfoods for allergies

Superfoods can play a key role in the management of food allergies. Ingredients such as turmeric, coconut oil, blueberries, and flaxseed offer specific benefits that help soothe allergy symptoms and improve a dog's overall health.

- **Turmeric**: Thanks to curcumin, it has natural anti-inflammatory properties that are ideal for reducing itching and reddening of the skin.
- **Coconut Oil**: Moisturizes dry skin and relieves itching, as well as supporting the immune system.
- **Flaxseed**: Provides omega-3s, useful for reducing inflammation and improving coat and skin health.
- **Blueberries**: Rich in antioxidants, they boost the immune system and fight oxidative stress.

Example: a stew of salmon, brown rice and carrots, enhanced with a teaspoon of coconut oil and a sprinkling of turmeric, can be a delicious and highly beneficial meal for a dog with allergies.

Specific recipes for common allergies

If your dog is allergic to chicken, beef or dairy products, it is essential to replace these ingredients with safe alternatives. For example:

- **For chicken allergies**: Use turkey, fish or lamb. A simple recipe might include steamed turkey, brown rice and broccoli.
- **For wheat or corn allergies**: Replace grains with sweet potatoes or quinoa. A delicious combination might be cooked lamb, boiled sweet potatoes and cooked spinach.

Managing cereal or lactose intolerances

For grain-intolerant dogs, you can create meals based on sweet potatoes, pumpkin and peas, avoiding wheat, barley or oats altogether. These alternative carbohydrates provide energy without causing digestive upset.

For lactose intolerance, avoid dairy products such as butter, milk or traditional cheeses. If necessary, you can use lactose-free natural yogurt or coconut milk to enrich some recipes.

Example: a porridge made with coconut milk, mashed banana and a sprinkling of chia seeds is a great breakfast for a dog with lactose intolerance.

Supplement safe and nutrient-rich vegetables

Vegetables are essential in a balanced diet, especially for dogs with allergies. Vegetables such as zucchini, carrots, spinach and broccoli are rich in fiber and vitamins and generally well tolerated. To improve digestibility, always steam or boil vegetables, removing any tough skins.

Example: a stew with turkey, zucchini, and sweet potatoes, with an addition of ground flaxseed, is a complete and easy-to-digest meal.

Monitoring and adapting recipes

Each dog is unique, and what works for one may not be suitable for another. After introducing a new recipe, watch carefully for any symptoms of allergy or intolerance, such as itching, diarrhea, or lethargy. If you notice adverse reactions, discontinue use of the suspect ingredient immediately and consult a veterinarian.

Plan meals and consult your veterinarian

Finally, to ensure a balanced diet, always consult a veterinarian or pet nutritionist. Planning meals in advance allows you to make sure your dog gets all the essential nutrients without risk. This approach will also help you save time and maintain a stable feeding routine for your dog.

With a carefully planned and customized diet, you can significantly improve your four-legged friend's health and quality of life by providing safe, nutritious and tasty meals.

LOW-FAT RECIPES

Low-fat diets are essential for dogs suffering from problems such as pancreatitis, obesity or specific metabolic conditions. These recipes are designed to provide a balanced, nutritious meal without overloading your dog's digestive system. By using lean protein, easily digestible carbohydrates, and fiber-rich vegetables, you can create tasty meals that support your four-legged friend's overall health and well-being.

1. Turkey and brown rice

Ingredients:

- **200g / 7,05oz lean ground turkey**
- **50g / 1,76oz cooked brown rice**
- **1 medium carrot**: Grated.
- **500ml / 0,13gal unsalted vegetable broth**

Preparation:

1. **Cook the turkey**: In a nonstick skillet, cook the turkey without adding oil, stirring until it is fully cooked.
2. **Combine the ingredients**: Add the cooked turkey, brown rice, and grated carrot to the vegetable broth.
3. **Final** cooking: Let simmer for 10 minutes.

2. Cod fillet with sweet potatoes

Ingredients:

- **150g / 5,30oz of cod fillet**
- **100g / 3,53oz sweet potatoes**: Peeled and diced.
- **50g / 1,76oz zucchini**: Cut into rounds.

Preparation:

1. Cook cod: Steam the cod fillet until tender.
2. **Prepare the vegetables**: Steam sweet potatoes and zucchini until soft.
3. **Combine**: Mix cod with cooked vegetables.

3. Chicken and pumpkin

Ingredients:

- **150g / 5,30oz chicken breast**: Cut into strips.
- **50g / 1,76oz cooked and mashed pumpkin**
- **1 tablespoon of puffed rice**

Preparation:

1. **Cook the chicken:** Grill the chicken without oil until fully cooked.
2. **Mix the ingredients together**: Combine the cooked chicken, crushed pumpkin, and puffed rice.

4. Turkey and Sspinach

Ingredients:

- **200g / 7,05oz ground turkey**
- **1 handful fresh spinach**: Chopped.
- **50g / 1,76oz potatoes**: Cut into cubes.

Preparation:

1. **Cook the turkey:** Cook the turkey in a nonstick pan.
2. **Prepare the vegetables**: Steam the potatoes and spinach.
3. **Combine**: Mix turkey with cooked vegetables.

5. White fish and carrots

Ingredients:

- **150g / 5,30oz white fish fillet (cod or hake)**
- **1 medium carrot**: Cut into rounds.
- **50g / 1,76oz cooked brown rice**

Preparation:

1. **Cook the fish:** Steam the fish.
2. **Prepare the vegetables**: Steam carrots until soft.
3. **Assemble the dish**: Mix the fish with the carrots and rice.

6. Turkey and peas

Ingredients:

- **200g / 7,05oz ground turkey**
- **50g / 1,76oz peas**: Fresh or frozen.
- **1 medium potato**: Cut into cubes.

Preparation:

1. **Prepare the ingredients**: Cook the turkey in a pan and steam the vegetables.
2. **Combine**: Combine turkey with peas and potato.

7. Chicken and zucchini

Ingredients:

- **150g / 5,30oz chicken breast**: Cut into small pieces.
- **50g / 1,76oz zucchini**: Cut into rounds.
- **50g / 1,76oz cooked brown rice**

Preparation:

1. **Cook the chicken**: Cook the chicken in a pan.
2. **Preparing** the zucchini: Steam the zucchini.
3. **Assemble**: Mix the chicken with the rice and zucchini.

8. Turkey and broccoli

Ingredients:

- **200g / 7,05oz ground turkey**
- **50g / 1,76oz broccoli**: Divided into florets.
- **50g / 1,76oz of sweet potatoes**

Preparation:

1. **Prepare the ingredients**: Cook the turkey in a pan and steam the vegetables.
2. **Stir**: Compose the dish by combining the ingredients.

9. Cod and zucchini

Ingredients:

- **150g / 5,30oz of cod fillet**
- **50g / 1,76oz zucchini**: Cut into rounds.
- **50g / 1,76oz of puffed rice**

Preparation:

1. **Prepare the ingredients**: Steam the cod and zucchini.
2. **Assemble**: Mix it all together with the puffed rice.

10. Chicken and carrots

Ingredients:

- **150g / 5,30oz chicken breast**
- **1 medium carrot**: Grated.
- **50g / 1,76oz cooked brown rice**

Preparation:

1. **Cook the chicken:** Grill the chicken.
2. **Assemble**: Mix the chicken with the rice and grated carrot.

11. Salmon and sweet potatoes

Ingredients:

- **150g / 5,30oz salmon fillet**: Remove any bones.
- **100g / 3,53oz sweet potatoes**: Peeled and diced.
- **50g / 1,76oz peas**: Fresh or frozen.

Preparation:

1. **Prepare the salmon**: Steam the salmon until tender.
2. **Cook vegetables**: Steam sweet potatoes and peas until soft.
3. **Combine**: Mix shredded salmon with cooked vegetables.

12. Turkey and pumpkin

Ingredients:

- **200g / 7,05oz ground turkey**
- **100g / 3,53oz pumpkin**: Cooked and pureed.
- **50g / 1,76oz cooked brown rice**

Preparation:

1. **Cook the turkey:** Cook the turkey in a nonstick pan without oil.
2. **Assemble**: Mix the cooked turkey with the pumpkin puree and rice.

13. White fish and spinach

Ingredients:

- **150g / 5,30oz of cod fillet**
- **1 handful fresh spinach**: Chopped.
- **50g / 1,76oz potatoes**: Cut into cubes.

Preparation:

1. **Cook the fish and potatoes**: Steam the cod and potatoes.

2. **Add spinach:** Add spinach in the last few minutes of cooking.

3. **Combine:** Mix all ingredients together.

14. Chicken and broccoli

Ingredients:

- **150g / 5,30oz chicken breast**
- **50g / 1,76oz broccoli**: Divided into florets.
- **50g / 1,76oz carrots**: Cut into rounds.

Preparation:

1. **Cook the** chicken: Grill the chicken or steam it.

2. **Cook vegetables**: Steam the broccoli and carrots.

3. **Assemble**: Mix the shredded chicken with the cooked vegetables.

15. Turkey and zucchini

Ingredients:

- **200g / 7,05oz ground turkey**
- **50g / 1,76oz zucchini**: Cut into rounds.
- **50g / 1,76oz of puffed rice**

Preparation:

1. **Cook the turkey:** Cook the turkey in a nonstick pan.

2. **Preparing** the zucchini: Steam the zucchini.

3. **Combine**: Mix cooked turkey, zucchini, and puffed rice.

16. Lamb and potatoes

Ingredients:

- **200g / 7,05oz of lean lamb**
- **100g / 3,53oz potatoes**: Peeled and diced.
- **50g / 1,76oz carrots**: Cut into rounds.

Preparation:

1. **Cook the lamb:** Cook the lamb in a nonstick pan.

2. **Cook vegetables**: Steam the potatoes and carrots.

3. **Assemble**: Mix the lamb with the cooked vegetables.

17. Cod and peas

Ingredients:

- **150g / 5,30oz of cod fillet**
- **50g / 1,76oz peas**: Fresh or frozen.
- **50g / 1,76oz cooked brown rice**

Preparation:

1. **Cook the cod:** Steam the cod.
2. **Cook peas**: Steam peas until tender.
3. **Combine**: Mix shredded cod with peas and rice.

18. Chicken and pumpkin

Ingredients:

- **150g / 5,30oz chicken breast**
- **100g / 3,53oz pumpkin**: Cooked and pureed.
- **50g / 1,76oz cooked brown rice**

Preparation:

1. **Cook the chicken:** Steam or grill the chicken.
2. **Assemble**: Mix the shredded chicken with the pumpkin puree and rice.

19. Turkey and carrots

Ingredients:

- **200g / 7,05oz ground turkey**
- **50g / 1,76oz carrots**: Cut into rounds.
- **50g / 1,76oz of sweet potatoes**

Preparation:

1. **Prepare** the turkey: Cook the turkey in a pan.
2. **Cook Vegetables**: Steam carrots and sweet potatoes.
3. **Assemble**: Mix all ingredients together.

20. White fish and broccoli

Ingredients:

- **150g / 5,30oz of cod fillet**
- **50g / 1,76oz broccoli**: Divided into florets.
- **50g / 1,76oz sweet potatoes**: Cut into cubes.

Preparation:

1. **Cook fish and vegetables**: Steam cod, broccoli and sweet potatoes.
2. **Combine**: Mix all ingredients to create a balanced meal.

These 20 recipes are designed to provide low-fat meals suitable for dogs with special needs. Each dish is easy to prepare, balanced and made with fresh ingredients to ensure maximum taste and nutritional value. Experiment with these combinations and customize them to your dog's preferences!

MENU FOR DOGS THAT ARE ELDERLY OR HAVE JOINT PROBLEMS

Older dogs or dogs with joint problems need specific nutrition that promotes joint health, reduces inflammation and supports mobility. Recipes for this category of dogs focus on nutrient-rich ingredients, such as lean protein, healthy fats, and superfoods with anti-inflammatory properties, such as turmeric, fish oil, and flaxseed. Here are 20 easy-to-prepare recipes to ensure a balanced and tasty diet for your dog.

1. Chicken, sweet potatoes and broccoli

Ingredients:

- **150g / 5,30oz chicken breast**: Cut into cubes.
- **100g / 3,53oz sweet potatoes**: Peeled and diced.
- **50g / 1,76oz broccoli**: Divided into florets.

Preparation:

1. **Cook chicken:** Steam or pan cook chicken without oil.
2. **Cook vegetables:** Steam sweet potatoes and broccoli until soft.
3. **Assemble:** Mix the chicken with the cooked vegetables and serve.

2. Turkey, brown rice and spinach

Ingredients:

- **200g / 7,05oz ground turkey**
- **50g / 1,76oz cooked brown rice**
- **1 handful of fresh spinach**

Preparation:

1. **Prepare** the turkey: Cook the turkey in a nonstick pan without oil.
2. **Cook spinach**: Add spinach in the last 2 minutes of cooking the turkey.
3. **Assemble**: Mix it with the cooked rice.

3. Salmon, quinoa and carrots

Ingredients:

- **150g / 5,30oz salmon**: Remove any bones.
- **50g / 1,76oz of cooked quinoa**
- **1 medium carrot**: Grated.

Preparation:

1. **Cook** the salmon: Steam the salmon until tender.
2. **Prepare** the quinoa: Cook the quinoa according to the instructions on the package.
3. **Combine**: Mix salmon with quinoa and grated carrot.

4. Chicken, squash and peas

Ingredients:

- **150g / 5,30oz chicken breast**
- **50g / 1,76oz pumpkin**: Cooked and pureed.
- **50g / 1,76oz peas**

Preparation:

1. **Cook the chicken:** Steam or pan cook the chicken.
2. **Prepare the ingredients**: Steam the peas and prepare the pumpkin puree.
3. **Assemble**: Mix all ingredients together.

5. Turkey, sweet potatoes and turmeric

Ingredients:

- **200g / 7,05oz ground turkey**
- **100g / 3,53oz sweet potatoes**: Cut into cubes.
- **1 pinch of turmeric**

Preparation:

1. **Cook the turkey:** Cook the turkey in a pan without oil.
2. **Cook sweet potatoes**: Steam them until they are soft.

3. **Combine**: Mix it all together and add a pinch of turmeric.

6. Cod, broccoli and zucchini.

Ingredients:

- **150g / 5,30oz of codfish**
- **50g / 1,76oz broccoli**: Divided into florets.
- **50g / 1,76oz zucchini**: Cut into rounds.

Preparation:

1. **Cook the cod:** Steam the cod.
2. **Prepare vegetables**: Steam broccoli and zucchini.
3. **Assemble**: Mix all ingredients together.

7. Chicken, brown rice and flaxseed

Ingredients:

- **150g / 5,30oz of chicken**
- **50g / 1,76oz cooked brown rice**
- **1 teaspoon ground flaxseed**

Preparation:

1. **Cook the chicken:** Cook the chicken in a pan or steam it.
2. **Assemble**: Mix cooked chicken with rice and add flaxseed.

8. Turkey, pumpkin and spinach

Ingredients:

- **200g / 7,05oz ground turkey**
- **50g / 1,76oz cooked pumpkin**
- **1 handful of fresh spinach**

Preparation:

1. **Prepare** the turkey: Cook the turkey in a pan.
2. **Assemble**: Mix the cooked turkey with the squash and spinach.

9. Salmon, sweet potatoes and peas

Ingredients:

- **150g / 5,30oz salmon**
- **100g / 3,53oz sweet potatoes**: Cut into cubes.
- **50g / 1,76oz peas**

Preparation:

1. **Cook the salmon:** Steam the salmon.
2. **Prepare ingredients**: Steam sweet potatoes and peas.
3. **Assemble**: Mix it all together to create a balanced meal.

10. Chicken, broccoli and brown rice

Ingredients:

- **150g / 5,30oz chicken breast**
- **50g / 1,76oz broccoli**: Divided into florets.
- **50g / 1,76oz cooked brown rice**

Preparation:

1. **Prepare** the chicken: Grill or cook the chicken.
2. **Cook broccoli**: Steam it.
3. **Assemble**: Mix the chicken with the broccoli and rice.

11. Cod, spinach and quinoa

Ingredients:

- **150g / 5,30oz cod fillet**: Remove any bones.
- **50g / 1,76oz of cooked quinoa**
- **1 handful of fresh spinach**

Preparation:

1. **Cook cod:** Steam cod until tender.
2. **Cook the quinoa**: Follow the instructions on the package to achieve a fluffy consistency.
3. **Add spinach**: Steam the spinach in the last few minutes.
4. **Assemble**: Mix the shredded cod with the quinoa and spinach.

12. Turkey, carrots and brown rice

Ingredients:

- **200g / 7,05oz ground turkey**
- **50g / 1,76oz cooked brown rice**
- **1 medium carrot**: Grated.

Preparation:

1. **Cook the** turkey: Brown the turkey in a nonstick pan.
2. **Prepare** the rice: Cook the rice and let it cool.
3. **Assemble**: Mix the turkey with the rice and add the grated carrot.

13. Chicken, peas and sweet potatoes

Ingredients:

- **150g / 5,30oz chicken breast**
- **50g / 1,76oz peas**: Fresh or frozen.
- **100g / 3,53oz sweet potatoes**: Cut into cubes.

Preparation:

1. **Prepare** the chicken: Steam or grill the chicken without oil.
2. **Cook vegetables**: Steam peas and sweet potatoes until soft.
3. **Assemble**: Mix the shredded chicken with the cooked vegetables.

14. Salmon, broccoli and sweet potatoes

Ingredients:

- **150g / 5,30oz salmon**: Remove any bones.
- **50g / 1,76oz broccoli**: Divided into florets.
- **100g / 3,53oz of sweet potatoes**

Preparation:

1. **Cook the salmon:** Steam the salmon.
2. **Prepare the vegetables:** Steam the broccoli and sweet potatoes.
3. **Assemble:** Mix the shredded salmon with the cooked vegetables.

15. Turkey, zucchini and brown rice

Ingredients:

- **200g / 7,05oz ground turkey**
- **50g / 1,76oz zucchini**: Cut into rounds.
- **50g / 1,76oz cooked brown rice**

Preparation:

1. **Prepare** the turkey: Cook the turkey in a nonstick pan without oil.
2. **Cook zucchini:** Steam zucchini until soft.
3. **Assemble**: Mix the cooked turkey with the rice and zucchini.

16. Chicken, pumpkin and spinach

Ingredients:

- **150g / 5,30oz of chicken breast**
- **50g / 1,76oz pumpkin**: Cooked and pureed.
- **1 handful of fresh spinach**

Preparation:

1. **Cook the chicken:** Steam or grill the chicken.
2. **Preparing the spinach**: Steam the spinach.
3. **Assemble**: Mix the shredded chicken with the pumpkin puree and spinach.

17. Cod, sweet potatoes and zucchini

Ingredients:

- **150g / 5,30oz of cod fillet**
- **100g / 3,53oz sweet potatoes**: Peeled and diced.
- **50g / 1,76oz of zucchini**

Preparation:

1. **Cook the cod:** Steam the cod.
2. **Cook vegetables**: Cook steamed sweet potatoes and zucchini.
3. **Assemble**: Mix it all together to create a balanced meal.

18. Turkey, spinach and puffed rice

Ingredients:

- **200g / 7,05oz ground turkey**
- **1 handful of fresh spinach**
- **50g / 1,76oz of puffed rice**

Preparation:

1. **Cook the turkey:** Cook the turkey in a nonstick pan.
2. **Preparing the spinach**: Steam the spinach.
3. **Assemble**: Mix the cooked turkey with the spinach and puffed rice.

19. Chicken, carrots and brown rice

Ingredients:

- **150g / 5,30oz chicken breast**
- **50g / 1,76oz carrots**: Cut into rounds.
- **50g / 1,76oz cooked brown rice**

Preparation:

1. **Preparing** the chicken: Steam or grill the chicken.
2. **Cook carrots**: Steam carrots until soft.
3. **Assemble**: Mix the chicken with the rice and carrots.

20. Salmon and brown rice with zucchini

Ingredients:

- **150g / 5,30oz salmon**
- **50g / 1,76oz cooked brown rice**
- **50g / 1,76oz zucchini**: Cut into rounds.

Preparation:

1. **Cook the salmon:** Steam the salmon.
2. **Preparing** the zucchini: Steam the zucchini.
3. **Assemble**: Mix the salmon with the rice and zucchini.

These additional recipes complement the menu for older dogs or dogs with joint problems, providing balanced, nutritious meals that support mobility, reduce inflammation, and promote optimal health. You can alternate these combinations to vary your dog's diet, ensuring that you always provide delicious, healthy meals for your dog.

9. SNACKS AND TREATS FOR SPECIAL OCCASIONS

HOMEMADE COOKIES: PUMPKIN SNACKS

Making homemade cookies for your dog is a great idea to provide a tasty and healthy snack. Pumpkin is a versatile and nutritious ingredient, rich in fiber, vitamin A and antioxidants, making it perfect for dogs of all ages. In this section, you will find 20 original pumpkin snack recipes, ideal for treating your four-legged friend to special occasions or just to let him know how much you love him.

1. Classic pumpkin cookies

Ingredients:

- **200g / 7,05oz pumpkin puree**: Fresh or canned, no sugar or spices.
- **150g / 5,30oz of whole wheat flour**
- **1 egg**

Preparation:

1. **Mix the ingredients together**: Combine pumpkin puree, flour and egg in a bowl. Mix until a firm dough forms.
2. **Shape the cookies**: Roll out the dough and cut out the desired shapes.
3. **Bake:** Bake at 180°C / 356°F for 20-25 minutes, until cookies are golden brown.

2. Pumpkin and apple cookies

Ingredients:

- 200g / 7,05oz of pumpkin puree
- 1 grated apple
- 150g / 5,30oz of oatmeal

Preparation:

1. **Prepare** the dough: Mix the pumpkin, apple and flour until smooth.
2. **Shape the cookies**: Cut the dough into small circles or bones.
3. **Bake:** Bake at 180°C / 356°F for 25 minutes.

3. Pumpkin and carrot cookies

Ingredients:

- 200g / 7,05oz of pumpkin puree
- 1 grated carrot
- 150g / 5,30oz of whole wheat flour

Preparation:

1. **Prepare the dough**: Mix the pumpkin with the carrot and flour.
2. **Shape cookies**: Create fun shapes such as bones or hearts.
3. **Bake**: Bake at 180°C / 356°F for 20 minutes.

4. Pumpkin and oatmeal cookies

Ingredients:

- 200g / 7,05oz of pumpkin puree
- 150g / 5,30oz of rice flour
- 50g / 1,76oz of oats

Preparation:

1. **Prepare the dough**: Combine pumpkin, flour and oats in a bowl.
2. **Shape the cookies**: Shape the dough into small discs.
3. **Bake:** Bake at 180°C / 356°F for 20 minutes.

5. Pumpkin and turmeric cookies

Ingredients:

- 200g / 7,05oz of pumpkin puree
- 1 pinch of turmeric
- 150g / 5,30oz of whole wheat flour

Preparation:

1. **Prepare the dough**: Mix the pumpkin, turmeric and flour.
2. **Shape the cookies**: Create rectangular shapes.
3. **Bake:** Bake at 180°C / 356°F (350°F) for 25 minutes.

6. Pumpkin and flaxseed cookies.

Ingredients:

- 200g / 7,05oz of pumpkin puree
- 1 tablespoon ground flaxseed
- 150g / 5,30oz of rice flour

Preparation:

1. **Prepare the dough**: Combine the ingredients in a bowl and mix.
2. **Shape the cookies**: Shape into small discs or bones.
3. **Bake**: Bake at 180°C / 356°F for 20-25 minutes.

7. Pumpkin and banana cookies

Ingredients:

- 200g / 7,05oz of pumpkin puree
- 1 ripe banana: Mashed.
- 150g / 5,30oz of oatmeal

Preparation:

1. **Prepare the dough**: Mix mashed banana with pumpkin and flour.
2. **Shape cookies**: Create round shapes.
3. **Bake**: Bake at 180°C / 356°F for 20 minutes.

8. Pumpkin and spinach cookies

Ingredients:

- **200g / 7,05oz of pumpkin puree**
- **1 handful fresh spinach**: Chopped.
- **150g / 5,30oz of rice flour**

Preparation:

1. **Prepare the dough**: Mix pumpkin, spinach and flour.
2. **Shape the cookies**: Create discs or bones.
3. **Bake**: Bake at 180°C / 356°F for 20 minutes.

9. Pumpkin and sweet potato cookies

Ingredients:

- **200g / 7,05oz of pumpkin puree**
- **100g / 3,53oz sweet potatoes**: Cooked and mashed.
- **150g / 5,30oz of whole wheat flour**

Preparation:

1. **Prepare the dough**: Mix pumpkin, sweet potatoes and flour.
2. **Shape the cookies**: Create rectangular shapes.
3. **Bake**: Bake at 180°C / 356°F (350°F) for 25 minutes.

10. Pumpkin and coconut oil cookies.

Ingredients:

- **200g / 7,05oz of pumpkin puree**
- **1 tablespoon of coconut oil**
- **150g / 5,30oz of whole wheat flour**

Preparation:

1. **Prepare the dough**: Combine all ingredients in a bowl.
2. **Shape the cookies**: Create round shapes.
3. **Bake**: Bake at 180°C / 356°F for 20 minutes.

11. Pumpkin and yogurt cookies

Ingredients:

- 200g / 7,05oz of pumpkin puree
- 1 tablespoon sugar-free natural yogurt
- 150g / 5,30oz of rice flour

Preparation:

1. **Prepare the dough**: Mix the pumpkin, yogurt and flour until smooth.
2. **Shape the cookies**: Cut the dough into small circles or fun shapes.
3. **Bake**: Bake at 180°C / 356°F for 20-25 minutes, until cookies are golden brown.

12. Pumpkin and blueberry cookies

Ingredients:

- 200g / 7,05oz of pumpkin puree
- 50g / 1,76oz fresh or frozen blueberries
- 150g / 5,30oz of whole wheat flour

Preparation:

1. **Prepare the dough**: Mix the pumpkin with the blueberries and flour.
2. **Shape the** cookies: Create small, flat cookies for easy baking.
3. **Bake**: Bake at 180°C / 356°F for 25 minutes.

13. Pumpkin and apple cookies

Ingredients:

- 200g / 7,05oz of pumpkin puree
- 1 medium apple: Grated.
- 150g / 5,30oz ground oats

Preparation:

1. **Prepare the dough**: Combine the pumpkin, grated apple and oats.
2. **Shape the cookies**: Shape them into small oval shapes.
3. **Bake**: Bake at 180°C / 356°F for 20 minutes.

14. Pumpkin and peanut butter cookies.

Ingredients:

- 200g / 7,05oz of pumpkin puree
- 1 tablespoon of natural peanut butter (no sugar or salt)
- 150g / 5,30oz of oatmeal

Preparation:

1. **Prepare the dough**: Mix pumpkin and peanut butter, then add flour.
2. **Shape the cookies**: Cut the dough into fun shapes.
3. **Bake:** Bake in the oven at 180°C / 356°F for 20-25 minutes.

15. Pumpkin and cinnamon cookies

Ingredients:

- 200g / 7,05oz of pumpkin puree
- 1 pinch of cinnamon
- 150g / 5,30oz of rice flour

Preparation:

1. **Prepare the dough**: Mix pumpkin, cinnamon and flour.
2. **Shape the cookies**: Roll out the dough and cut out shapes.
3. **Bake**: Bake at 180°C / 356°F for 20 minutes.

16. Pumpkin and sunflower seed cookies.

Ingredients:

- 200g / 7,05oz of pumpkin puree
- 1 tablespoon unsalted sunflower seeds
- 150g / 5,30oz of whole wheat flour

Preparation:

1. **Prepare the dough**: Mix the pumpkin with the sunflower seeds and flour.
2. **Shape the cookies**: Create small round cookies.
3. **Bake**: Bake at 180°C / 356°F for 25 minutes.

17. Pumpkin and potato cookies

Ingredients:

- 200g / 7,05oz of pumpkin puree
- 100g / 3,53oz boiled potatoes: Mashed.
- 150g / 5,30oz of whole wheat flour

Preparation:

1. **Prepare the dough**: Mix the pumpkin with the mashed potatoes and flour.
2. **Shape the cookies**: Shape into rectangular or round shapes.
3. **Bake**: Bake at 180°C / 356°F for 25 minutes.

18. Pumpkin and spinach cookies

Ingredients:

- 200g / 7,05oz of pumpkin puree
- 1 handful fresh spinach: Finely chopped.
- 150g / 5,30oz of rice flour

Preparation:

1. **Prepare the dough**: Mix the pumpkin with the spinach and flour.
2. **Shape the cookies**: Create thin disks or other shapes.
3. **Bake**: Bake at 180°C / 356°F for 20-25 minutes.

19. Pumpkin and banana cookies

Ingredients:

- 200g / 7,05oz of pumpkin puree
- 1 ripe banana: Mashed.
- 150g / 5,30oz of oatmeal

Preparation:

1. **Prepare the dough**: Combine pumpkin and banana, then add flour.
2. **Shape the cookies**: Cut the dough into small circles or oval shapes.
3. **Bake**: Bake at 180°C / 356°F for 20 minutes.

20. Pumpkin and ginger cookies.

Ingredients:

- 200g / 7,05oz of pumpkin puree
- 1 pinch of grated ginger
- 150g / 5,30oz of whole wheat flour

Preparation:

1. **Prepare the dough**: Mix pumpkin, ginger and flour until smooth.
2. **Shape the cookies**: Create small rectangular or round shapes.
3. **Bake**: Bake in the oven at 180°C / 356°F for 20-25 minutes.

Each recipe is designed to be simple to prepare and adaptable to your four-legged friend's specific needs, ensuring a delicious and nutritious snack for any special occasion.

TREATS FOR BIRTHDAYS AND HOLIDAYS

Homemade treats for your dog's birthday or holiday are a special way to show love and care by providing a festive snack that is both tasty and healthy. By using dog-safe ingredients and simple recipes, you can create desserts and treats suitable for any celebration. Here are 10 recipes ideal for celebrating with your four-legged friend.

1. Pumpkin banana cake

Ingredients:

- 200g / 7,05oz of pumpkin puree
- 1 ripe banana: Mashed.
- 150g / 5,30oz of whole wheat flour
- 1 egg

Preparation:

1. **Prepare the dough**: Mix the pumpkin, banana, egg and flour until smooth.
2. **Bake the cake**: Pour the batter into a muffin tin or small cake pan.
3. **Bake**: Bake at 180°C / 356°F for 25 minutes. Let cool before serving.

2. Peanut butter cookies for holidays

Ingredients:

- 200g / 7,05oz of whole wheat flour
- 2 tablespoons of natural peanut butter (no sugar or salt)
- 1 egg

Preparation:

1. **Prepare the dough**: Mix the flour, peanut butter and egg until a firm dough forms.
2. **Shape the cookies**: Cut out the dough with Christmas or birthday-themed shapes.
3. **Bake**: Bake at 180°C / 356°F for 20 minutes.

3. Apple and cinnamon cupcakes

Ingredients:

- 150g / 5,30oz of rice flour
- 1 grated apple
- 1 teaspoon cinnamon powder
- 100ml / 0,03gal of water

Preparation:

1. **Prepare the dough**: Mix the grated apple, cinnamon, flour and water until it forms a thick mixture.
2. **Fill ramekins**: Pour batter into paper or silicone ramekins.
3. **Bake**: Bake at 180°C / 356°F for 20 minutes.

4. Banana and yogurt ice cream

Ingredients:

- **2 ripe bananas**: Frozen and cut into pieces.
- 100g / 3,53oz of sugar-free natural yogurt

Preparation:

1. **Blend the ingredients**: Blend frozen bananas and yogurt until creamy.
2. **Freeze**: Pour the mixture into popsicle molds and freeze for 2-3 hours.
3. **Serve**: Remove the ice creams from the molds and offer them to your dog as a refreshing treat.

5. Pumpkin and blueberry tarts

Ingredients:

- 200g / 7,05oz of pumpkin puree
- 50g / 1,76oz fresh or frozen blueberries
- 150g / 5,30oz of whole wheat flour

Preparation:

1. **Prepare** the dough: Mix the flour with a little water to create a solid dough.
2. **Create the tarts**: Line small molds with the dough and fill them with the pumpkin puree and blueberries.
3. **Bake**: Bake at 180°C / 356°F for 20-25 minutes.

6. Christmas cookies with honey and cinnamon

Ingredients:

- 200g / 7,05oz of whole wheat flour
- 1 tablespoon of honey
- 1 pinch of cinnamon

Preparation:

1. **Prepare the dough**: Mix all the ingredients together until you have a firm mixture.
2. **Shape cookies**: Create Christmas shapes such as stars or little trees.
3. **Bake**: Bake at 180°C / 356°F for 20 minutes.

7. Sweet potato pancakes

Ingredients:

- 150g / 5,30oz cooked and mashed sweet potatoes
- 1 egg
- 50g / 1,76oz of oatmeal

Preparation:

1. **Prepare the dough**: Mix sweet potatoes, egg and flour until smooth.
2. **Cook pancakes**: Pour small amounts of batter onto a hot nonstick skillet and cook on both sides until golden brown.
3. **Serve**: Let cool before serving to your dog.

8. Birthday Turkey Cake

Ingredients:

- **200g / 7,05oz ground turkey**
- **100g / 3,53oz sweet potatoes**: Cooked and mashed.
- **50g / 1,76oz fresh spinach**: Chopped.

Preparation:

1. **Prepare** the mixture: Mix the turkey, sweet potatoes and spinach in a bowl.
2. **Bake the cake**: Pour the mixture into a baking dish and bake at 180°C / 356°F (350°F) for 30 minutes.
3. **Decorate**: Let cool and decorate with a few grated carrots.

9. Birthday Carrot Cookies.

Ingredients:

- **150g / 5,30oz grated carrots**
- **150g / 5,30oz of whole wheat flour**
- **1 egg**

Preparation:

1. **Prepare the dough**: Mix carrots, flour and egg until smooth.
2. **Forming cookies**: Use themed shapes to create fun cookies.
3. **Bake**: Bake at 180°C / 356°F for 20 minutes.

10. Pumpkin and peanut butter muffins.

Ingredients:

- **200g / 7,05oz of pumpkin puree**
- **1 tablespoon of natural peanut butter**
- **150g / 5,30oz of oatmeal**

Preparation:

1. **Prepare the dough**: Mix all ingredients until thick.
2. **Fill ramekins**: Pour batter into muffin molds.
3. **Bake**: Bake in the oven at 180°C / 356°F for 20-25 minutes.

These recipes not only add a special touch to your dog's celebrations, they are also safe and healthy. Personalize each treat with edible dog decorations or fun shapes, and turn any occasion into an unforgettable celebration!

HOW TO PREPARE HEALTHY AND SAFE SNACKS

Making healthy and safe snacks for your dog is a loving gesture that allows you to be in full control of the ingredients and meet your four-legged friend's specific needs. Homemade snacks are free of the additives, preservatives and artificial sugars often found in industrial products. In addition, they can be customized to suit any allergies, intolerances or food preferences your dog may have. Below we explore strategies and tips for creating tasty, nutritious, and safe snacks.

Select Quality Ingredients

The choice of ingredients is critical to ensure the safety and nutritional value of snacks. Opt for fresh, organic and dog-friendly foods. Lean proteins, such as chicken, turkey, and fish, are great for protein-rich snacks. Carbohydrates such as sweet potatoes and brown rice provide energy, while vegetables such as carrots, zucchini, and spinach add vitamins and fiber.

Example: **Chicken and Carrot Snack**

- Steam 200g / 7,05oz chicken breast and 100g / 3,53oz carrots. Whisk together to make a thick paste, shape it into small patties and bake at 180°C / 356°F for 20 minutes.

Avoid Toxic or Dangerous Foods

When preparing snacks for your dog, avoid ingredients that can be harmful. These include chocolate, onion, garlic, grapes, raisins, xylitol and spicy spices. Also make sure that any bones used are well cooked and not chippable.

Example: **Banana Oatmeal Cookies**

- Mix 1 mashed banana, 100g / 3,53oz oats and 50 ml water. Create small, flat cookies, then bake at 180°C / 356°F for 20 minutes.

Use Superfood for Extra Benefits

Superfoods such as flaxseed, turmeric, blueberries, and coconut oil can be added to enhance the nutritional value of snacks. These ingredients provide antioxidants, essential fatty acids and anti-inflammatory properties that support the dog's overall health.

Example: **Turmeric patties**

- Mix 200g / 7,05oz ground turkey with a pinch of turmeric and 50g / 1,76oz chopped spinach. Shape patties and bake at 180°C / 356°F for 25 minutes.

Adapting Recipes to Your Dog's Needs

Every dog is unique, and snacks should be tailored to his size, age, activity level and health status. For older dogs or dogs with dental problems, create snacks that are soft and easy to chew. For puppies or active dogs, choose snacks rich in protein and energy.

Example: **Sweet Potato Energy Bars**

- Mix 150g / 5,30oz cooked sweet potato, 100g / 3,53oz oats and 1 tablespoon natural peanut butter. Spread the mixture on a baking sheet, cut into bars and bake at 180°C / 356°F for 25 minutes.

Safe Snack Preparation

Safe preparation is crucial to avoid contamination or storage problems. Always wash your hands, use clean utensils, and make sure ingredients are fresh. Avoid adding salt or sugar to snacks and cook them completely to eliminate any bacteria.

Example: **Pumpkin and Chia Seed Cookies**

- Mix 200g / 7,05oz pumpkin puree, 1 tablespoon chia seeds and 150g / 5,30oz rice flour. Create cookies and bake at 180°C / 356°F for 20 minutes.

Control Portions and Frequency

Snacks, however healthy, should only be a small part of your dog's diet. Offer them as a treat or snack, avoiding exceeding 10 percent of the daily calorie intake. Adjust the size of snacks according to your dog's size.

Example: **Salmon Mini Snack**

- Blend 150g / 5,30oz steamed salmon with 50g / 1,76oz sweet potatoes. Shape small balls and bake at 180°C / 356°F for 15 minutes.

Experiment with Shapes and Ingredients

Snacks can be made more fun by using themed cookie cutters or colorful, safe ingredients. For example, use grated carrots for an orange twist or spinach for bright green. This also makes them perfect for special occasions.

Example: **Colorful Beet Cookies**

- Mix 100g / 3,53oz beet puree, 200g / 7,05oz whole wheat flour and 50 ml water. Cut out the dough with star shapes and bake at 180°C / 356°F for 20 minutes.

Frozen Snacks for Hot Days

During the summer, make refreshing and hydrating snacks using frozen ingredients such as natural yogurt, fruits and vegetables. These snacks are easy to prepare and perfect for keeping your dog fresh.

Example: **Watermelon and Yogurt Cubes**

- Blend 200g / 7,05oz seedless watermelon with 100g / 3,53oz natural yogurt. Pour mixture into ice molds and freeze for 2 hours.

Storage of Snacks

Homemade snacks must be stored properly to maintain freshness. Store cookies in an airtight container for up to 5 days, or freeze them to extend their shelf life. Soft snacks should be refrigerated and eaten within 3 days.

Example: **Chicken and Spinach Chunks**

- Mix 150g / 5,30oz chopped cooked chicken, 50g / 1,76oz spinach and 50g / 1,76oz puffed rice. Shape into balls and refrigerate for up to 3 days.

Involve Your Dog

Making homemade snacks can be a fun activity for the whole family. Let your dog "witness" the preparation and let him smell the ingredients, creating a unique time of sharing.

Example: **Apple Cinnamon Cookies**

- Mix 100g / 3,53oz grated apple, 1 pinch cinnamon and 150g / 5,30oz oatmeal. Create cookies and bake at 180°C / 356°F for 20 minutes.

Preparing healthy and safe snacks for your dog is not only a loving gesture, but also an opportunity to offer him something truly special and nutritious. With a little creativity and attention to ingredients, you can turn every snack into a moment of joy and well-being.

10 TIPS TO SAVE TIME AND BUDGET

HOW TO PLAN MEALS FOR THE WEEK

Planning your dog's meals for the entire week is not only an effective way to save time and money, but also a strategy to ensure that your dog's diet remains balanced and nutritious. With careful planning, you can optimize ingredients, reduce waste, and make sure your dog gets all the nutrients he needs. Here is a detailed guide to organizing your dog's weekly meals in a practical and sustainable way.

Establish a Weekly Plan

The first step to effective planning is to create a detailed weekly plan. This helps you visualize your dog's meals for each day, balancing sources of protein, carbohydrates, vegetables and healthy fats. Use a table or spreadsheet to record meals, including snacks and treats, so you have a complete picture of the diet.

Example:

- **Monday:** Turkey, sweet potatoes, spinach.
- **Tuesday:** chicken, brown rice, carrots.
- **Wednesday:** Cod, quinoa, zucchini.
- **Thursday:** Turkey, potatoes, broccoli.
- **Friday:** Salmon, brown rice, spinach.

- **Saturday:** Chicken, sweet potatoes, peas.
- **Sunday:** turkey, carrots, brown rice.

Prepare in Advance

Devoting one day a week to meal preparation is an excellent way to save time. Cook large quantities of food, divide them into daily portions and store them in airtight containers. Store portions for the first three days in the refrigerator and freeze those for the rest of the week. This way, you will always have fresh, ready-to-eat meals on hand.

Practical tip:

Prepare a common base of rice or sweet potatoes and combine it with different proteins to vary the weekly menu.

Choose Versatile and Affordable Ingredients

Opt for ingredients that can be used in different combinations to create variety without complicating your life. For example, turkey can be combined with sweet potatoes and spinach in one meal, or with brown rice and zucchini in another. This strategy reduces costs and allows you to make the best use of purchased ingredients.

Example:

- **Turkey:** Use it in stews or as a main protein.
- **Carrots:** Add them raw as snacks or cooked in main meals.
- **Sweet Potatoes:** Use them as a base for energy dishes or as a sweet and nutritious addition.

Organize the Pantry and Freezer

Keeping a well-organized pantry and freezer is essential for effective planning. Store dry ingredients, such as rice, oats and flour, in airtight labeled containers. In the freezer, divide raw protein into portions suitable for your dog and freeze them immediately to preserve freshness.

Pro   tip:

Freeze unsalted broth in small cubes to add to weekly meals as a source of flavor and hydration.

Prepare Multipurpose Recipes

Creating recipes that can be easily adapted or reused is a great way to save time. For example, a large stew of turkey, sweet potatoes, and carrots can be served as is on a day, or used as a filling for homemade snacks or combined with rice for a different meal.

Example:

- **Basic Stew:** Cook 500g / 17,64oz turkey, 300g / 10,58oz sweet potatoes and 200g / 7,05oz carrots in unsalted broth.

- **Variant 1:** Serve with a sprinkling of flax seeds.
- **Variant 2:** Add 100g / 3,53oz of brown rice for a complete meal.

Balance the Nutrients

Make sure each meal contains a balanced combination of protein, carbohydrates and vegetables. A balanced diet supports your dog's health and reduces the risk of nutritional deficiencies. If necessary, consult a veterinarian or pet nutritionist to ensure that the weekly schedule meets your dog's specific needs.

Example of proportions:

- **Protein:** 50% of the meal (chicken, turkey, fish).
- **Carbohydrates:** 25 percent of the meal (sweet potatoes, brown rice).
- **Vegetables:** 25 percent of the meal (spinach, zucchini, carrots).

Use Tools to Save Time

Appliances such as slow cookers, pressure cookers, or food processors can greatly simplify meal preparation. A slow stove, for example, allows you to cook large quantities of food with minimal effort. Simply add all the ingredients in the morning and have the meals ready for portioning in the evening.

Example:

- **Recipe for Slow Cooker:** Put 500g / 17,64oz chicken, 300g / 10,58oz sweet potatoes, 200g / 7,05oz carrots and 1 liter / 0,26gal unsalted broth in the slow cooker. Cook at a low temperature for 6-8 hours.

Monitor and Adapt the Plan

Each dog has unique dietary needs, so it is important to monitor how he or she reacts to the weekly plan and make changes if necessary. If you notice your dog is hungry between meals, consider increasing portions or adding healthy snacks. On the other hand, if your dog seems to be gaining weight, reduce the amount of carbohydrates slightly.

Planning meals for your dog is a habit that takes some practice, but the benefits in terms of time saved, budget optimized, and your furry friend's health are enormous. With a little organization, useful tools and quality ingredients, you can create an efficient system that will make your dog's meals not only healthy and balanced, but also easy for you to manage.

SMART SHOPPING: CHEAP AND QUALITY INGREDIENTS

When it comes to preparing meals for your dog, choosing inexpensive but high-quality ingredients is essential to keeping the household budget in check without compromising your four-legged friend's health. With a little planning and care, you can find nutritious and affordable ingredients that are a perfect fit for your dog's diet. Here are some practical tips for shopping smart and getting the most out of your budget.

Know Your Dog's Nutritional Needs.

Before you start shopping, it is critical to understand what your dog needs for a balanced diet. Lean protein, complex carbohydrates and nutrient-rich vegetables should be the basis of every meal. Choose ingredients that provide sustainable energy and support overall health, such as chicken, turkey, brown rice and carrots, which are often available at affordable prices.

Take advantage of Deals and Buy in Quantity

One way to save money is to buy basic ingredients in large quantities. For example, brown rice and oats can be bought in large bags at a very low cost per serving. Similarly, proteins such as chicken and turkey often cost less when purchased in family packages or directly from a local butcher. You can freeze excess portions for future use, thus reducing waste.

Opt for Seasonal Vegetables

Seasonal vegetables not only taste better but are also cheaper than out-of-season vegetables. For example, in autumn, squash and sweet potatoes are plentiful and inexpensive, while in spring carrots, zucchini, and spinach are readily available. Use these vegetables as the basis for your dog's meals, combining them with protein and carbohydrates.

Choose Cheap Meat Cuts

Not all cuts of meat are equal in cost, but many cheaper cuts are perfect for your dog's diet. For example, bone-in chicken, ground turkey, or beef for stew are generally less expensive than higher-quality cuts. Slow cooking these cuts makes them tender and easy for your dog to digest.

Example:

- **Chicken Stew**: Slow cook bone-in chicken pieces along with sweet potatoes and carrots in a pressure cooker or slow cooker. Remove bones before serving.

Evaluate Frozen or Chilled Ingredients.

Frozen ingredients are often cheaper and just as nutritious as fresh ones. Frozen peas, spinach and blueberries are great options to add to your dog's meals. In addition, you can find competitively priced frozen meat and fish that are ideal for planning weekly meals.

Buy Directly from Local Producers

Supporting local farmers and butchers not only allows you to get fresh ingredients, but often at a lower price than supermarkets. You can ask for deals on less popular cuts of meat or buy bulk vegetables directly from local markets.

Home Preparation to Save Money

Making snacks and meals for your dog at home is generally cheaper than buying industrial food. With simple ingredients such as whole wheat flour, natural peanut butter and carrots, you can make healthy cookies at a fraction of the cost of commercial products.

Example:

- **Rice and Pumpkin Cookies**: Mix 200g / 7,05oz pumpkin puree with 150g / 5,30oz rice flour. Shape cookies and bake at 180°C / 356°F for 20 minutes.

Avoid Waste and Reuse Leftovers

Leftover lean meat, cooked vegetables, and simple carbohydrates such as rice and potatoes can be reused to create meals for your dog. Make sure leftovers do not contain seasonings, salt or toxic ingredients such as onions and garlic. This approach not only reduces waste but also saves you money.

Compare Prices and Make Shopping List

Before shopping, compare prices at different stores and supermarkets. A well-organized shopping list will help you stay focused and avoid unnecessary spending. Put only essential ingredients, such as protein, carbohydrates, and vegetables, on the list.

Experiment with Cheap Recipes

Finally, use simple, inexpensive recipes that you can vary with the ingredients you have on hand. For example, a turkey stew with sweet potatoes can be modified by adding zucchini or spinach, depending on what you find on offer.

Example:

- **Turkey Stew**: Cook ground turkey with sweet potatoes, carrots and unsalted broth. Serve as a complete meal or freeze in portions.

With these tips, you can create a healthy, balanced and economical diet for your dog while saving time and money. Shopping smart doesn't mean sacrificing quality: with a little planning and creativity, you can provide your dog with nutritious and tasty meals without breaking your budget.

BATCH PREPARATION: SAVES TIME WITHOUT COMPROMISING QUALITY

Preparing your dog's meals in batches is a smart strategy to save time, reduce stress, and ensure that your four-legged friend always has healthy, balanced meals available. With a well-organized approach, you can cook a substantial amount of food at one time, divide it into portions, and store it for future use. Here's how to implement this technique without sacrificing quality.

Planning Lots

Before you start cooking, create a plan for weekly or biweekly meals. Decide which recipes to prepare and how many meals you need to cover the entire period. For example, if your dog eats twice a day, you will need 14 meals for a week. Choose 2-3 main recipes to alternate, thus ensuring variety and nutritional balance.

Example plan:

- **Lot 1**: Turkey with sweet potatoes and zucchini.
- **Lot 2**: Chicken with brown rice and carrots.
- **Lot 3**: Cod with quinoa and broccoli.

Preparation of Ingredients

Preparing ingredients in advance is essential to speed up the cooking process. Wash, peel and chop all vegetables, and divide proteins into suitable portions. Use different containers for each ingredient to maintain order during preparation.

Suggestion:

- Cut vegetables into uniform pieces to ensure even cooking.
- Separate raw proteins according to recipes to avoid confusion.

Cooking in Large Quantities

Take advantage of large pots, slow cookers or pressure stoves to cook large quantities of food. These tools allow you to cook multiple portions evenly and simultaneously. For example, a turkey and vegetable stew can be prepared in a slow cooker while cooking brown rice in a separate pot.

Example:

- **Chicken and Carrot Stew**: Put 500g / 17,64oz chicken, 300g / 10,58oz carrots, 200g / 7,05oz sweet potatoes and 1 liter / 0,26gal unsalted broth in a slow cooker. Cook at a **low temperature** for 6 to 8 hours.

Portioning and Storage

Once the food is ready, divide it into daily portions or per meal. Use airtight containers for storage in the refrigerator or freezer. Make sure each container contains an adequate amount for one meal, thus avoiding waste and simplifying daily management.

Suggestion:

- Use clear containers and label them with the date of preparation and contents.
- Freeze portions that you will not use within 2-3 days.

Maximizes Variety

Even with batch preparation, it is important to ensure some variety in your dog's meals. Alternate recipes throughout the week and experiment with different ingredients, such as quinoa, fish or spinach. This not only keeps your dog interested in the food, but also provides a wider range of essential nutrients.

Example of variation:

- A batch of chicken with sweet potatoes and carrots can be alternated with turkey, zucchini and brown rice.

Reduce Waste

Batch preparation helps you use ingredients more efficiently, reducing food waste. For example, if you buy a large package of carrots, you can use them in several recipes throughout the week. Also, you can reuse leftover vegetables to make unsalted broths to use as a base for future meals.

Practical tip:

- Save the stems and peels of vegetables such as carrots or zucchini to make homemade broths.

Optimize Time with Appropriate Tools

Using tools such as food processors, food choppers, and digital scales can greatly speed up preparation. For example, a food processor can chop vegetables in seconds, while a digital scale helps you measure portions accurately, ensuring balanced meals.

Quality Monitoring

Even with batch preparation, it is important to keep the quality of meals high. Always use fresh ingredients, check food expiration dates, and ensure that frozen food is used within the recommended safe period (generally within 3 months).

Weekly Preparation Routine

Establishing a routine for batch meal preparation simplifies the process and makes it sustainable over time. Dedicate one fixed day a week to cooking, portioning, and organizing meals. Over time, this routine will become an integral part of your daily management.

Batch preparation not only saves you valuable time, it also ensures that your dog gets nutritious, well-balanced meals every day. With a little organization and proper tools, you can maximize your time in the kitchen and devote more energy to quality time with your furry friend.

CONCLUSION

REFLECTING ON THE JOURNEY OF HOME COOKING FOR DOGS

Embarking on the journey of home cooking for your dog is more than just a change in eating routine-it is an act of love and dedication that strengthens the bond between you and your four-legged friend. Through meal preparation, you have the opportunity to directly influence your dog's health and well-being by providing him with nutritious, tasty food tailored to his specific needs. Reflecting on this journey, we can examine the lessons learned, the benefits gained, and the intrinsic value of this choice.

Preparing homemade food for your dog takes time, planning and a certain amount of creativity, but the benefits are obvious. Not only do you have complete control over the ingredients used, but you can also closely monitor how each change in the diet affects your dog's health. This level of individualized attention is impossible to achieve with prepackaged commercial food.

For example, many owners report that, with a home-cooked diet, their dogs show visible improvements in coat health, increased energy, and smoother digestion. For a dog with special dietary needs, such as allergies or food sensitivities, home cooking can be a life-saving solution.

One of the most rewarding aspects of cooking for your dog is the ability to customize each meal. Every dog is unique, with specific tastes, preferences, and needs. Maybe your dog loves chicken but is less enthusiastic about fish, or maybe he prefers vegetables like carrots and zucchini over spinach. With home cooking, you can experiment with different combinations and continually adapt meals.

For example, if your dog suffers from arthritis, you can include ingredients such as turmeric or fish oil for their anti-inflammatory properties. If he needs more energy, you can increase the amount of complex carbohydrates, such as sweet potatoes or brown rice. Each food choice becomes a conscious gesture to support your dog's health.

Although preparing homemade meals may seem like a more onerous commitment than buying kibble or packaged wet food, it is important to consider it as an investment in your dog's health. Food-related diseases, such as obesity, diabetes, or gastrointestinal problems, can be prevented or mitigated through a healthy, balanced diet. Reducing the risk of these conditions not only improves your dog's quality of life, but can also result in long-term veterinary cost savings.

For example, a dog fed a balanced homemade food will be less likely to develop dental, digestive or weight problems. In addition, a diet rich in antioxidants, vitamins and minerals can support the immune system, helping it fight infections and diseases.

Cooking for your dog is not just about nutrition-it is also a way to strengthen the bond between you. Mealtime becomes a shared experience in which your dog feels pampered and appreciated. Food preparation, with your dog watching you slice vegetables or mix ingredients, creates a sense of anticipation and happiness. This simple but meaningful gesture builds mutual trust and affection.

Many owners report that, through home cooking, they develop a deeper understanding of their dog's preferences and reactions. This not only improves the dog's quality of life, but also makes the relationship with the owner richer and more meaningful.

The journey of home cooking for dogs is full of lessons and discoveries. You've probably learned more about the ingredients, portions, and essential nutrients needed for your dog's well-being. You may have faced a few early mistakes, such as overly large portions or less successful ingredient combinations, but each challenge has helped hone your ability to feed your dog optimally.

In addition, you developed practical skills, such as using tools like slow cookers or digital scales to ensure accuracy and time savings. You discovered the importance of batch planning and preparation, turning what might have seemed like a challenging task at first into a manageable routine.

The transition to home cooking for your dog often leads to increased awareness for your own and your family's diet as well. By learning to select fresh ingredients, avoid additives, and balance meals, you may have developed a new perspective on the importance of healthy, natural eating.

This holistic approach to nutrition can inspire a healthier lifestyle for the whole family by promoting better eating habits and reducing the use of processed foods.

Looking ahead, the future of home cooking for dogs offers endless possibilities. You can continue to experiment with new recipes, discover local or seasonal ingredients, and learn more about your dog's nutritional needs. If you feel particularly inspired, you could even share your experience with other dog owners by offering suggestions or organizing times to share ideas and recipes.

In addition, the growing interest in natural pet food is prompting many manufacturers to offer specific high-quality ingredients, making it easier for owners to adopt this food choice.

Ultimately, home cooking for dogs is not just a practical act, but a tangible expression of the love you have for your four-legged companion. Every meal you prepare is an opportunity to care for his well-being and happiness. It is a commitment that brings with it a deep satisfaction, knowing that you are doing everything you can to provide your dog with a long, healthy and joyful life.

Reflecting on this journey, it is clear that home cooking for dogs is much more than a food trend-it is an act of connection, awareness, and love that enriches the lives of both of you. With each meal you prepare, you are building a bright and healthy future for your furry friend, making each day together even more special.

A HEALTHY AND HAPPY FUTURE FOR YOUR DOG

Offering your dog a healthy and happy future is every loving owner's dream. Having embarked on the journey of home cooking, you have already taken a vital step toward this goal. But a prosperous future depends on more than just nutrition-it's an intertwined set of factors, from caring for your dog's physical and mental health to caring for his environment and relationships. In this final reflection, we'll explore how to build a bright future for your dog of love, well-being, and satisfaction.

The basis for a long and healthy life is a balanced and nutritious diet. Home cooking allows you to provide tailored meals that meet your dog's unique needs. However, nutrition is not a static process. As your dog ages, he may have different needs: puppies require foods rich in protein and calcium to promote growth, while older dogs may benefit from diets with ingredients that support joints and immune systems.

For example, an older dog with joint problems might benefit from meals enriched with turmeric and fish oil, while a young, active dog may require larger portions and nutrient dense to maintain his energy.

Tip:

Consult a veterinarian regularly to update your dog's food plan based on his age, weight, and activity level.

In addition to nutrition, your dog's physical well-being requires regular exercise, veterinary visits, and good hygiene. Daily walks, interactive games and training sessions not only keep your dog fit but also strengthen the bond between the two of you. In addition, regular checkups at the vet help you prevent or manage any health problems early on.

For example, incorporating activities such as swimming can be helpful for dogs with joint problems, while searching games stimulate the mind and burn energy for young, active dogs.

A healthy dog is also a mentally stimulated dog. Boredom can lead to undesirable behaviors such as biting furniture or excessive barking. Incorporating activities that stimulate the mind, such as dog puzzles, hide-and-seek games or advanced training, keeps your dog engaged and satisfied.

Pro tip:

Create personalized toys using safe materials you have around the house. For example, fill a container with homemade kibble and let your dog look for it.

Your dog's happy future depends not only on what you do for him, but also on the quality of the relationships he builds. Socializing your dog, exposing him to different environments, people and other animals, is essential for his emotional balance. A well-socialized dog is more confident, less anxious, and happier.

For example, take your dog to dedicated parks, enroll both of you in obedience classes or arrange to meet other dogs to create positive interaction experiences.

Your dog lives in the environment you create for him. Provide him with a space that is safe, clean and full of stimulation. This includes a comfortable kennel, appropriate toys and regular access to open spaces. If you live in an apartment, make sure he has enough opportunities to exercise and interact with the outdoors.

For example, regular toy rotations or creating new "adventures" around the house, such as an obstacle course, can keep your dog involved and happy.

Life is full of changes, and your dog relies on you to face them with confidence. Whether it is a move, the arrival of a new family member, or a change in routine, the key to ensuring a peaceful future is to prepare your dog for the change. Introduce new things gradually and patiently, maintaining a stable routine as much as possible.

For example, if you are planning a move, take your dog to the new home for short visits before the final move so that he gets used to it gradually.

As technology and scientific knowledge continue to advance, the future offers more and more opportunities to improve your dog's life. Health-monitoring apps, training devices, and the use of genetic testing to prevent specific diseases are just some of the resources that could help you offer your dog a better life.

For example, using a dog GPS tracker can help you monitor your dog's activity levels, ensuring that he gets the exercise he needs each day.

Finally, the best way to ensure a healthy and happy future for your dog is to appreciate every moment together. From meal preparation to daily walks, each shared activity strengthens your bond and creates precious memories. Remember that your dog lives in the present, and the time you spend with him is the greatest gift you can give him.

With a combination of balanced nutrition, exercise, mental stimulation and lots of love, you can create a bright future for your dog. Every little gesture, from choosing ingredients for meals to spending time playing, contributes to his overall well-being. By reflecting on everything you have learned and done for your four-legged friend, you can be sure that you are giving your dog not only a healthy life, but also one filled with happiness and love.

INVITATION TO SHARE YOUR JOURNEY

Home cooking for dogs is much more than a food choice: it is a personal journey of discovery, experimentation and moments of connection with your four-legged friend. Like any journey, it becomes even more meaningful when it is shared. Recounting your experience can not only inspire other owners to embark on a similar journey, but it also provides an opportunity to learn from others, building a community that puts the well-being of dogs first.

Why Share Your Path?

Sharing your expertise in home cooking for dogs is not simply about showing off your favorite recipes. It is a way to create awareness about the importance of healthy, natural food for pets. Many owners may not know the benefits of home cooking or think it is too complicated. Your story can demonstrate how doable it is, as well as highlight the tangible benefits to your dog's health and happiness.

For example, telling how you have seen improvements in your dog's digestion, energy level, or coat quality from a homemade diet can be a powerful motivator for other owners.

Sharing Through Social Media

Social media is an amazing platform for sharing your journey. You can post photos of the meals you prepare, tell anecdotes about your dog, and even share simple recipes that other owners can try. A post on Instagram, a video on YouTube, or an article on a personal blog can reach a large community of pet lovers.

Pro tip:

- Use specific hashtags such as #CookingHousesForDogs or #RecipesForDogs to make your content easy to find.
- Also share mistakes and lessons learned: they show authenticity and help others avoid the same obstacles.

Join Online Groups and Forums

Many people seek support and ideas in pet-related groups and forums. By joining these communities, you can share your experience and learn from others. Forums such as Reddit or Facebook groups dedicated to dog care are great places to discuss recipes, planning strategies, and achievements.

Example:

- If you have found that a certain ingredient has improved your dog's health, please share this information and ask others to share their experiences.

Organize Local Events or Meetings

If you feel particularly involved, you can take your experience offline. Arrange meetings with other dog owners in your area to exchange ideas, cook together, or simply discuss the benefits of home cooking. These meetings can become an opportunity to build meaningful relationships and raise awareness about animal health.

Suggestion:

- Bring printed recipes or make small homemade snacks to share with other participants.

Sharing to Receive Feedback

Sharing your journey is not only a way to inspire others, but also to receive feedback and new ideas. Home cooking for dogs is an ever-evolving field, and every contribution can enrich your knowledge. Someone might suggest an ingredient you've never considered or a more efficient method of preparation.

For example, you may find that others use alternative flours, such as chickpea or coconut, to create gluten-free snacks, expanding your dog's meal options.

Inspiring a New Generation of Owners

Your example can be especially valuable to new dog owners, who often find themselves overwhelmed by all the decisions they have to make. By sharing your journey, you can show them that providing healthy nutrition is not only possible, but also rewarding. Your experience can become a reference point for those who are at the beginning of this adventure.

Creating an Archive of Recipes and Tips

One of the most useful forms of sharing is to create an organized archive of your recipes and practical tips. This can be a simple document shared online, a personal blog, or even a small ebook collecting best practices and tested recipes. By offering this tool, you can help other owners save time and get started with confidence.

The Impact of Sharing

When you share your journey, you contribute to a broader movement toward greater awareness of the importance of good pet nutrition. Each post, conversation, or meeting can inspire another owner to make a positive change in their dog's life.

For example, you may not realize how much your story can influence someone who is looking for a solution to their dog's health problems. Your experience may become the impetus they need to start home cooking and improve another dog's quality of life.

Sharing your journey in home cooking for dogs is an act of generosity and passion. It is a way to amplify the impact of your choices, helping others discover the benefits of healthy, natural eating. In every recipe shared, in every tip offered, is the potential to make a significant difference. Don't underestimate the power of your story-it could inspire many others to take the same path, creating a community united by a love of dogs and care for their well-being.

APPENDIX

TABLE OF NUTRITIONAL VALUES OF INGREDIENTS

Below you will find a table listing the nutritional values of the ingredients used in the proposed recipes, with the data referring to 100g / 3,53oz of product (1g corresponds to 0.04 oz), 10kcal = 41,87kJ. These values will help you better understand the nutritional content of the foods used for your dog's home diet.

Ingredient	Calories (kcal)	Protein (g)	Fats (g)	Carbohydrates (g)	Fiber (g)	Notes
Chicken Breast	165	31.0	3.6	0.0	0.0	Source of lean protein, ideal for supporting muscle growth.
Ground Turkey	135	27.0	3.0	0.0	0.0	Versatile protein that is easy to digest.
Cod Fillet	82	18.0	0.7	0.0	0.0	Rich in protein and low in fat, perfect for dogs with food sensitivities.
Salmon	208	20.0	13.0	0.0	0.0	Rich in omega-3s, good for healthy skin and coat.
Sweet Potatoes	86	1.6	0.1	20.1	3.0	Source of complex carbohydrates, rich in vitamin A.
Brown Rice	111	2.6	0.9	23.0	1.8	Digestible carbohydrate, provides long-term energy.
Quinoa	120	4.1	1.9	21.3	2.8	Contains all essential amino acids, excellent plant protein source.
Carrots	41	0.9	0.2	9.6	2.8	Rich in vitamin A, useful for vision and the immune system.
Zucchini	17	1.2	0.3	3.1	1.0	Hypocaloric and rich in water, perfect for hydrating and providing fiber.
Spinach	23	2.9	0.4	3.6	2.2	Source of iron, calcium and antioxidants.

Ingredient	Calories (kcal)	Protein (g)	Fats (g)	Carbohydrates (g)	Fiber (g)	Notes
Pumpkin	26	1.0	0.1	6.5	0.5	Highly digestible, helps intestinal health.
Peas	81	5.4	0.4	14.5	5.7	Rich in fiber and plant protein.
Apple	52	0.3	0.2	13.8	2.4	Provides quick energy, contains vitamin C.
Banana	89	1.1	0.3	22.8	2.6	Rich in potassium and easily digestible carbohydrates.
Turmeric	354	7.8	9.9	64.9	21.0	Natural anti-inflammatory, use in small amounts.
Linseed	534	18.3	42.2	28.9	27.3	Rich in omega-3 and fiber, they promote digestion.
Fish Oil	902	0.0	100.0	0.0	0.0	Concentrated source of omega-3, essential for coat and joint health.
Unsalted Broth	15	0.5	0.0	0.5	0.0	Ideal for hydrating meals and adding flavor without sodium.
Whole Wheat Flour	340	13.2	2.5	72.6	10.7	Rich in fiber, ideal for snacks and cookies.
Rice Flour	366	7.2	1.0	80.1	1.3	Gluten-free, easy-to-digest alternative.
Oats	389	16.9	6.9	66.3	10.6	Rich in fiber and protein, good for intestinal health.
Natural Yogurt	59	10.0	0.4	3.6	0.0	Source of calcium and probiotics, useful for digestion.
Blueberries	57	0.7	0.3	14.5	2.4	Rich in antioxidants, they support the immune system.

This table provides an overview of the main nutrients in the ingredients used in recipes. Use it as a reference to balance your dog's meals and make sure you are meeting his nutritional needs. Always remember to consult a veterinarian for any specific needs related to your four-legged friend's diet.

THANKS

The making of this book has been a journey of discovery and growth, made possible through the support and inspiration of many special people and creatures who have enriched each page.

First of all, I would like to thank my faithful four-legged companion, who inspired every recipe, every tip, and every word in this book. His joy in enjoying homemade meals and his infectious enthusiasm were the driving force that made this project possible.

Special thanks also go to the veterinarians and pet nutrition experts who guided me with their valuable advice. Their commitment and dedication to animal welfare enabled me to fully understand the importance of a balanced and healthy diet.

Deep appreciation goes to my family and friends, who encouraged me at every stage of this project. Thank you for testing some of the recipes (and no, I don't just mean the dogs!) and sharing valuable suggestions. Your trust and enthusiasm have sustained me even in the most challenging moments.

Thank you also to the readers and animal lovers who decided to embark on this journey with me. It is your love for your dogs and desire to offer them the best that inspired me to write this book. I hope you will find the recipes and tips shared here useful, and that they can help make the lives of your furry friends even happier and healthier.

Finally, a special thanks to all the dogs of the world, whose unconditional affection reminds us every day what it means to be loved without reservation. This book is dedicated to you and the joy you bring into our lives.

With gratitude and affection,

Zoey Harper

Made in the USA
Las Vegas, NV
18 March 2025